THE SUPERFOODS DIET GUIDE

PREVENTION'S

FAMILY HEALTH LIBRARY™

THE SUPERFOODS DIET GUIDE

The Best Foods and Key Vitamins for Better Health

by the Editors of
Prevention® Magazine

 Rodale Press, Emmaus, Pa.

Printed in the United States of America on recycled paper containing a high percentage of de-inked fiber.

Library of Congress Cataloging in Publication Data

The Superfoods diet guide.

    (Prevention's family health library)
    On t.p. the registered trademark symbol "TM" is superscript following "library" in ser. title.
    1. Nutrition. 2. Vitamins. 3. Health.
I. Prevention (Emmaus, Pa.) II. Series.
[DNLM: 1. Diet—popular works. 2. Nutrition—popular works. QU 145 S959]
RA784.S86   1987   613.2   86-31338
ISBN 0-87857-708-4   paperback

2 4 6 8 10 9 7 5 3 1 paperback

NOTICE

    This book is intended as a reference volume only, not as a medical manual or guide to self-treatment. If you suspect that you have a medical problem, we urge you to seek competent medical help. Keep in mind that nutritional and health needs vary from person to person, depending on age, sex, health status and total diet. The information here is intended to help you make informed decisions about your health, not as a substitute for any treatment that may have been prescribed by your doctor.

Contents

1. A Cornucopia of Superfoods 1

They range from peppers to poultry, beans to broccoli—and they're part of a shopping list that could make you healthier.

2. Spot Your Nutritional Danger Zones 8

Even seemingly balanced diets can have hidden deficiencies. Here's how to pinpoint yours.

3. Eating for One 15

Unfortunately, research shows that good nutrition rarely comes in single servings. But your diet doesn't have to suffer just because you live alone.

4. Getting Kids to Eat Right 21

Just when the need for good food is most critical, kids often develop self-destructive eating habits. Here, two knowledgeable nutritionists offer timely advice.

5. A Nutritional Strategy to Slow Aging 32

Here's exciting new evidence that diet can alter the devastating side effects of aging by strengthening the body's own defense system.

6. The Good Meats 37
Lean meats, muscled with nutrition power, don't have to be trimmed from your diet.

7. Getting the Most Out of the F Complex 41
Scientists are scrutinizing dietary fiber as never before—and discovering that it does more and is more than they ever guessed.

8. Your Heart, Your Health and a Drink or Two 48
Can moderate drinking actually be good for you? Nobody wants to say yes, yet.

9. The Health Scoop on Ice Cream 56
How does America's favorite desert compare nutritionally with other popular snack foods? The results may surprise you.

10. Coffee and You 62
You may be the best judge of whether you can drink coffee—and how much is too much.

11. Health-Rating America's Favorite New Foods 67
These popular edibles taste good, but how good for you are they?

12. See If You Need More C 74
Does your body have enough vitamin C protection? Don't answer until you take this quiz.

13. Give Yourself the Iron Test—and Rate Your Energy Reserves 79
This easy test will let you know whether your diet is iron rich or iron poor.

14. A Consumer's Guide to the Amazing Aminos 85
These protein components are the new "vitamins of the 80's." Here's the promise of new healing powers, and the cautions we must observe.

CHAPTER 1

A Cornucopia of Superfoods

There was a time when the phrase "health food" conjured up the image of a monastic meal with all the lip-smacking lusciousness of grass and moon dust.

Today, healthy foods have taken on a whole new mainstream meaning. No longer esoteric edibles available only in health-food stores, they're foods fresh from the supermarket and produce stand, superfoods that medical researchers believe really may make us healthy.

Their evidence? Healthy people like the Eskimos, whose snacks of whale blubber should make them prime candidates for heart disease before 40 but whose fish diet actually seems to protect their hearts from harm; Italy's Neapolitans, whose high-fiber, low-fat natural foods keep them fit; the Seventh-day Adventists, largely vegetarians, who serve up a menu for long life.

There's evidence from the laboratory too. Did you know there is a substance in cabbage and its clan that actually may "trap" cancer-causing agents in your body before they do any harm? Or that carrots, rich in beta-carotene, can decrease your risk of lung cancer? Or that something called a protease inhibitor found in seeds, beans and rice may actually be an antidote to the cancer-causing effects of a high-fat diet?

Like the medical researchers, we turn to the laboratory and to healthy people when we put together our own well-balanced menu of superfoods. We also filled in with some of the foods Mother Nature blessed with a cornucopia of nutrients, such as liver, oysters and green

1

and red peppers. To make shopping easier, we included foods that, with perhaps one exception, you can find in any supermarket. And we offer them now to you with a toast: To your health!

Amaranth

You might not find this little-known grain on your market shelves—yet. Amaranth is a food of the future. It is literally manna to the millions of malnourished people of the Third World because it is remarkably high in protein and lysine, an essential amino acid—far higher than any other cereal grain. It also contains significant amounts of iron and magnesium. And it's versatile. You can use its leaves in salad and its seed for breakfast cereal, snacks or flour for baking.

Bananas

The banana disputes the old theory that if something tastes good it can't be good for you. Bananas are a great-tasting source of potassium, vitamin B_6 and biotin, another B vitamin. A medium banana contains about 100 calories, making it a delicious snack or dessert for dieters.

Beans

If you don't know beans about beans, consider this: In several tests on patients with high blood lipids (a risk factor for heart patients), a bean diet brought down cholesterol and triglyceride levels significantly, with no serious side effects. Beans are also high in magnesium, a good heart mineral, and the B vitamins thiamine, B_6 and riboflavin. They're also an excellent nonmeat source of iron.

Bran

One researcher calls wheat bran "the gold standard" against which the other brans, like oat and corn, are measured. Well, these days the other two are measuring up just fine. In a study of the effects of bran on constipation, corn bran was found to be therapeutically superior to wheat bran, probably because corn bran is 92 percent fiber compared to wheat bran's 52 percent fiber. Another group of researchers, at the University of Texas Health Science Center, also found in a feeding study with rats that corn bran cereal, even though it contained sucrose, helped prevent cavities.

And oat bran has been found to lower cholesterol as much as 13 percent in studies done by James Anderson, M.D., and associates, at the Veterans Administration Medical Center in Lexington, Kentucky.

Cabbage and Its Clan

Broccoli, brussels sprouts and cauliflower all figure prominently in the anticancer diet prescribed by the National Academy of Sciences. They appear to have some cancer-fighting properties, including vitamin A. And a cooked stalk of broccoli alone has all the Recommended Dietary Allowance (RDA) of A and twice the RDA of vitamin C, another cancer fighter, as well as calcium and potassium. Cabbage, brussels sprouts and cauliflower contain a substance that has been shown to "trap" certain carcinogens before they damage the body. University of Minnesota researcher Lee Wattenberg, M.D., found that these vegetables enhance a natural detoxification system in the small intestine that keeps the carcinogen away from susceptible tissues.

Carrots

Carrots are very high in beta-carotene, a precursor of vitamin A that is associated with a decreased risk of cancer. High in fiber, low in calories, even the crunch in carrots is good, toning and strengthening the gums.

Citrus Fruits

A group of Florida researchers noticed that residents of southeastern Florida, many of whom have backyard citrus trees, have a lower incidence of colon and rectal cancers than people in the northern parts of the nation. The scientists at Florida Atlantic University in Boca Raton believe the secret is in the fruit. They say the vitamins A, C and E and pectin fiber have a synergistic effect that may prevent cancer.

Fish

Holy Mackerel! Would you believe you could lower your blood pressure and cholesterol and triglyceride levels by eating mackerel and salmon? Researchers worldwide have discovered that certain types of fish— those containing eicosapentanoic acid, a fatty acid—protect against heart disease. They were tipped off by the healthy hearts of Greenland Eskimos, whose diets were otherwise high in fat. Apparently, it's a special kind of fat, which researchers at the Oregon Health Sciences University say may be "metabolically unique" and useful in controlling other fats that can clog the bloodstream.

Garlic and Onions

Bad for your breath but wonderful for the rest of you. A spate of studies found these two odoriferous roots can lower your cholesterol and their oils inhibit tumor growth in the laboratory. Onions have been used to slow down platelet aggregation or clumping, which can lead to deadly blood clots.

Herbs and Spices

Before you throw away your saltshaker and sugar bowl, consider refilling them—with herbs and spices. They're actually more flavorful substitutes. A couple of dashes of curry powder on fresh roasted nuts or popcorn and you'll never miss the salt. And as for sweets, the American Spice Trade Association found that desserts and beverages with sugar and other sweeteners replaced by spices drew rave reviews from a panel of tasters. They even loved blueberry shortcake sweetened with fruit juice and cinnamon and creamy custard with reduced sugar and a surprising bay leaf added for sweetness.

Kale, Spinach and the Leafy Greens

Your mother—and the National Academy of Sciences—insist that you eat your leafy green vegetables. Here's why you should: Greens like spinach contain chlorophyll, a substance that helps plants turn sunlight into food. Chlorophyll also has been found to lower the tendency of cancer-causing agents to cause genetic damage to your body's cells. Spinach and the other greens also contain significant amounts of vitamin A and calcium, although their oxalic-acid content can change calcium into an indigestible compound in the body. Kale, on the other hand, has far more calcium than oxalic acid, so it's a good source of this bone-strengthening mineral.

Liver

Usually found smothered in another superfood, onions, beef liver contains almost every nutrient going. It's rich in iron, zinc, copper, vitamins A, E, K, thiamine, riboflavin, biotin, folate, B$_{12}$, choline and inositol. Who can ask for anything more?

Melons

Cantaloupes and honeydews are low calorie treats or high-energy breakfast sources of vitamin C. One two-inch wedge of honeydew, for example, has only 49 calories but supplies more than half the RDA of vitamin C.

Nuts

You can consume a considerable portion of your minimum daily requirement of zinc during an afternoon snack if you're snacking on nuts. Nuts, especially cashews and almonds, are very high in this trace mineral so necessary for cell growth. But don't go nutty with nuts. Zinc notwithstanding, you're also munching a handful of calories, so enjoy them in moderation.

Oysters

Legend has it that oysters are an aphrodisiac. We don't make any claims for that, but oysters are high in zinc, shown to be necessary for proper prostate and sexual functioning and sperm mobility. Oysters are also rich in calcium, iron, and copper and iodine. But a word of caution. You'll rarely hear us say this about anything else: Don't eat them raw. Oysters tend to pick up bacteria that can make you ill if they're not cooked.

Peppers

Which has more vitamin C, an orange or a pepper? Better bet on the pepper. One of these gorgeous green beauties contains twice the vitamin C of an orange. And an amazing thing happens when peppers age. They turn red—and fill up with a good supply of vitamin A.

Poultry

Let's talk turkey. And chicken while we're at it. They're low in calories, low in fat, high in essential nutrients and taste. An average half a chicken breast contains 25.7 grams of protein, just 5.1 grams of fat and only 160 calories. With that you get a side order of vitamin A, riboflavin and niacin, not to mention iron. A chicken leg contains only 88 calories and 3.8 grams of fat. Turkey is equally good news. Three ounces of light meat without skin totals 150 calories, 28 grams of protein and 3.3 grams of fat, with respectable amounts of B vitamins.

Seeds

High in zinc and protein, seeds (such as pumpkin, sunflower and sesame seeds) also contain something called a protease inhibitor, which seems to help protect us against cancer. Protease inhibitors have been shown to prevent liver, mammary and colon cancer in cancer-prone laboratory animals.

Soup

It's not only good food, it's the food that makes you eat less. A study that analyzed the food diaries of 90 patients determined that those who ate soup more than four times a week ate fewer calories a day and lost more weight than those who didn't eat as much soup. In fact, the researchers found, a soup meal contained an average of 54.5 percent fewer calories than a nonsoup meal.

Soybeans

They're good protein—as good as animal sources, say nutritionists at the Massachusetts Institute of Technology. They lower cholesterol, say researchers at Washington University School of Medicine. And there's some indication that soybeans are cancer fighters. Like seeds, soybeans contain protease inhibitors. And soybean products like tofu (bean curd) and miso (soybean paste) tested by researchers in Tokyo seemed to inhibit potential carcinogens called n-nitrosamines in the stomach.

Sprouts

They're more than just a grassy accoutrement to salad and sandwich. Studies show that the ascorbic acid (vitamin C) in some sprouted seeds and beans increases 29- to 86-fold after germination! Mung bean sprouts are especially high in magnesium and calcium. But the best news concerns the wheat sprout. It's been shown to inhibit the genetic damage to cells caused by some cancer-causing agents.

Sweet Potatoes

This superfood is a sleeper that deserves to appear on the dinner table at times other than Thanksgiving and Christmas. Besides being tastier than white potatoes—no relation—they're high in vitamin A, the substance that makes carrots such a potent cancer-fighter. Sweet potatoes are also low in calories. One five-inch potato contains only 148 calories.

Wheat Germ

The B vitamin thiamine is abundant in only a few foods. But one of them is wheat germ, which is also rich in vitamin B_6. This versatile food was one relegated to the breakfast table but is now being used in everything from breads to salads.

Whole Grains

A generation ago when the only place you could get a piece of good whole grain bread was at the health-food store or in the kitchen of a wise health-minded cook. Whether it's bread, cereal or brown rice, the whole grains are everywhere now. They're an excellent source of dietary fiber, suspected of protecting us from everything from cholesterol to cancer. A recent Welsh study found that people who ate wholemeal bread were less likely to die from cerebrovascular disease.

Yogurt

African Masai warriors eat large portions of fermented cow's milk daily, which makes their already low cholesterol levels drop even lower. In the United States, fermented cow's milk is marketed as yogurt and appears to have a similar effect on American cholesterol levels. When 26 people in a study at Vanderbilt University went on a diet of whole- and skim-milk yogurt, their cholesterol levels dropped significantly. Rich in calcium and all the nutrients in a glass of milk, yogurt is also easier to digest for people who are intolerant to plain milk.

CHAPTER 2

Spot Your Nutritional Danger Zones

Quick! What are the four basic food groups? What does romaine lettuce have that iceberg doesn't? How about brown rice over white? What foods are rich in magnesium? Potassium? Zinc? What's a healthy amount of fat to have in your diet? How about protein? Carbohydrates? And—take a guess—just how many "essential nutrients" are there, anyway? (Hint: You *won't* find the answer by counting the ingredients on a multivitamin bottle label.)

If you answered even the first question correctly (see the box at the end of this chapter), you're ahead of the crowd, some nutritionists say. And if you've got every one right, you're excused from class. You really know the details when it comes to nutrition, and if you use that knowledge to eat better, you can count yourself one of the lucky few.

Research shows many Americans are increasingly concerned about what's in the 1,500 pounds of food they chow down each year. They're eating fewer frankfurters, less luncheon meat, sugar and candy, oils and fats. They're eating more chicken, cheese, dark green vegetables and citrus fruits.

Their concern is certainly a step in the right direction, but most still have a way to go, says Paul LaChance, Ph.D., professor of nutrition and food science at Rutgers University in New Brunswick, New Jersey. "The average American doesn't know where the nutrients are. He doesn't go shopping and pick up a vegetable and say, 'Here's my vitamin A, or here's my vitamin C.' He'll read the label on a prepared food, but won't know what it means. When it comes to details, most people just don't know much about nutrition."

And they have misconceptions, contends Phyllis Havens, R.D., a Hampden, Maine, consulting nutritionist. "People think margarine is so much better than butter, but then they'll use twice as much of it, not realizing there's as much fat and calories in it as butter," she says. "And they think granola bars are a healthy snack, when they're actually loaded with fat and sugar."

Havens is "re-educating" the clients she sees in her private practice and at the Holistic Center in South Portland, using an updated version of the four basic food groups. "I am encouraging people to look at them again, as a guide, but with an emphasis on specific nutrients and whole foods—whole grains, low-fat dairy products, fresh fruits, dark green leafy vegetables, and fish and poultry."

It's often not just lack of knowledge, but certain patterns of eating, or even patterns of living, that predispose many of us to dietary problems. And these dietary problems can often turn into health problems. Let's look at several common eating patterns or diets and see what's wrong with each. Where are the hidden danger zones and how can they be eliminated?

The High-Protein Predicament

Jean and Jerry like the quick weight loss diet. It lets them fill up on their favorite foods—steak and shrimp—and still drop five pounds in a week. It also allows them to eat plenty of chicken, low-fat cheese, lean fish and hard-boiled eggs, and to drink as much diet soda and coffee as their kidneys can handle. It prohibits any other foods. No fruits or vegetables. No carbohydrates. It's a diet they go on again and again, every time they regain those five pounds.

What's wrong with this diet? For starters it's high in fat. Fifty percent or more of its calories come from fat. "Anyone who's worried about heart disease or liver or kidney problems would want to avoid eating this way," Dr. LaChance says. "And it's also higher in sodium than is wise."

Fiber in this diet would be minuscule. "You are begging for dependency on a laxative," Dr. LaChance says. Low fiber intake could aggravate gallstones or diverticulosis, Havens adds.

Such a diet might not deliver all the calcium you need, and its high protein content would make your body excrete up to twice the calcium it would normally. "Unless you are eating a lot of low-fat dairy products, you could definitely increase the risk of osteoporosis (thin, weak bones), especially for older women, with this diet," Havens says.

And all the other nutrients that are found mostly in fruits, vegetables and whole grains would be missing in this diet—vitamins C and A, magnesium, potassium, and, among the B complex, thiamine, B_6 and folate. "When you see the number of nutrients that aren't being delivered and the health risks involved, you have to ask yourself, 'Why should I use this diet?'" Dr. LaChance says.

Adding insult to injury, much of that exhilaratingly quick weight loss on the high-protein diet is water, water that gushes back into your body the minute you resume eating carbohydrates. Both nutritionists recommend a reducing diet high in fiber and low in fats. "I recommend a diet similar to the Pritikin Diet [high in grains and vegetables, very low in fat] but one that allows about 20 percent fat," Havens says. Dr. LaChance likes *The F-* [for fiber] *Plan Diet* (Crown Publishers). Both allow you ample quantities of food, while minimizing the most concentrated source of calories—fat.

The Iron Impasse

Let's look at another dieter, Joan, who's proud of her superslim figure and admits she practically lives on a few low-cal staples—cottage cheese, yogurt, broiled chicken and fish, lettuce and tomato, zucchini and string beans. She's also a big tea and coffee drinker. She thinks it helps dull her appetite. And it perks her up. Trouble is, she hasn't been feeling very perky lately.

Joan's big problem is iron. She's getting less than half of what she needs from her food, and her tea and coffee drinking further inhibits absorption of the little she does get, according to Havens.

"I would put the focus on lots of dark green leafy vegetables like broccoli, spinach and even some of the more unusual greens like collards, mustard and kale," she says. "And I would try to convince her that some iron-rich legumes like beans and lentils aren't all that fattening. A half cup of cooked kidney beans has only 110 calories."

Dr. LaChance is very concerned about the difficulty of absorbing iron from grains and vegetables. "I'd suggest instead some of the very lean red meats, the muscle meats from the shoulder and rump." Women unwilling to eat much red meat will have to take an iron supplement, he believes.

How about someone who's eating no meat at all? When they went vegetarian ten years ago, Tom and Tina had the best of intentions. They'd read Frances Moore Lappé's *Diet for a Small Planet* and shifted their preferences toward dairy products, eggs, grains and plenty of fresh fruits and vegetables. They even got to like tofu and miso. They were determined to avoid all the ills associated with an overabundant society—obesity, high blood pressure, heart disease. But were they setting themselves up for trouble?

Both zinc and iron deficiencies can be a problem in a vegetarian diet, especially for women, researchers have found. And vegans, who eat no dairy products or eggs, often get less than the Recommended Dietary Allowance for calcium. "No vegetable is a reliable souce of zinc, and I'm very supportive of every vegetarian taking a zinc supplement," Havens says.

"And I think it's worthwhile if they're not feeling the highest energy level possible to have a blood test to see if they are iron deficient." If they are, she will try adding iron-rich legumes, blackstrap molasses and dark green leafy vegetables to their diet for three months, then have a second blood test done. If the dietary changes aren't working, she'll then suggest an iron supplement.

Calcium may be less of a problem. A surprising source of calcium can be tofu, when set into curd with calcium carbonate, says Georgene Barte, associate professor of foods and nutrition at Oregon State University, Corvallis. One serving of tofu has about a third the amount of calcium a serving of milk has.

B_{12} used to be considered an inevitable deficiency for strict vegetarians. Now, though, researchers have found significant amounts of B_{12} in cultured and fermented foods like miso, soy sauce and tempeh.

Vegetarians should realize that hard cheeses and nuts can be much higher in fats than lean red meat. One ounce of Cheddar cheese has 9.1 grams of fat; one ounce of lean, trimmed T-bone steak, only 3 grams. An ounce of almonds (about 22 nuts) has 16.4 grams of fat.

"I think vegetarians are more likely to go overboard with fats when they first make the switch, when instead of eating meat, they are eating whole-milk dairy products and eggs," says Havens. "I'd avoid those 'gourmet' vegetarian cookbooks that emphasize sour cream, cheese and eggs."

How about someone whose problem is a vegetable aversion?

Meat Eater's Malaise

As far as Frank is concerned, the only vegetable "real men" eat is potatoes—french-fried with a burger, boiled with a pot roast, or hash-browned with eggs. Like the picky little kid he was, Frank finds most fruits and vegetables yucky. But his childish holdover could be making him deficient in vitamins A, E and folate, and potassium.

Let's not knock potatoes. A medium baked spud with skin has 944 milligrams of potassium (about a third of the usual daily adult intake), 30 milligrams of vitamin C (half the RDA) and four grams of fiber, about a third of what many people get in a day. The problem is in the way most of us cook potatoes, says Barte. We peel the nutrient- and fiber-rich skin off, and boil or fry away some of the vitamin C. Frank should be eating a baked potato, skin and all.

And adding even a few choice fruits and vegetables to his limited menu could make the difference between health and deficiency.

"I find that some adults who are really turned off by cooked vegetables do better with raw ones," says Havens. "If they don't like cooked spinach, I suggest they start eating it raw mixed in with iceberg lettuce, gradually increasing the amount. Or they might enjoy dips with carrots or green pepper strips."

Like many children, some adults dislike strong-flavored vegetables like cabbage, broccoli and onions. Instead, they may enjoy carrots, winter squash and sweet potatoes, served with a little butter and maple syrup. These vegetables would certainly solve Frank's vitamin A problem. A four-ounce serving of sweet potatoes or carrots would supply his RDA of 5,000 International Units (I.U.), as would a half cup of butternut squash. Citrus fruits and juices would be his best bet for vitamin C. One cup of orange juice would give him 124 milligrams of C, and an additional bonus of 496 milligrams of potassium and 500 I.U. of A.

Calcium Countdown

Mary's daughter has been nagging her to get more calcium in her diet ever since Mary broke her wrist in a fall a few years ago. Now she's 70 and unsteady on her feet. Her daughter fears she'll fall down and break a hip one of these days.

The problem is that Mary thinks she gets all the calcium she needs: a cup of milk a day, with cereal and coffee, and another serving as a slice of cheese or half a cup of cottage cheese. Other foods boost her daily intake to the RDA of 800 milligrams. But that amount is not enough to prevent osteoporosis, researchers say.

"From what I've read, I think the RDA for women past 30 should be 1,000 milligrams, and for those past menopause, 1,200 to 1,500 milligrams," says Barte.

Getting that much calcium in your diet would mean getting the equivalent of four or five cups of milk. Each cup has 290 milligrams of calcium or 34 milligrams per ounce. One big miscalculation is that people think one serving of cottage cheese, normally about a quarter cup, equals the calcium in a cup of milk. It actually takes about two cups of cottage cheese to equal one cup of milk, Barte says.

The only foods that top dairy products for calcium content are sardines and salmon, but only if you eat the soft small bones mixed in with the flesh. Sardines have 124 milligrams of calcium per ounce; salmon, 63 milligrams.

No Time for Nutrition

What if you're like Joan, concerned with getting an entire busy family to eat better? Both she and her husband work, and he's on the road a day or two each week. When her two teenage sons aren't in school, they're at band practice or a swimming meet. Joan gave up on sit-down meals when she realized the only family member willing to show up on a regular basis was the dog.

Now meals are whenever you're hungry and whatever you manage to scrounge out of the refrigerator. She tries to keep it stocked with foods the kids like and can easily fix themselves—ground beef, tuna, cheese, eggs, hot dogs and beans, bread, milk, cold cuts, frozen pizzas. And, of course, sodas, potato chips and ice cream. Her kids would mutiny if she didn't keep those things around the house. She's about the only one who eats the salad fixings she brings home. She'd like her family to eat better, but where to start?

The dangers in this diet are too much fat and sugar, and too little fiber, B and C vitamins, and minerals like magnesium and potassium, Havens says.

"If she were willing to commit even a few hours a week to cooking, she could make a huge pot of nutritious soup with beans, brown rice and all kinds of vegetables, keep part in the refrigerator and freeze some for use later. I do that myself, and I'm a busy professional."

Planning ahead by making and freezing large batches of other good foods—chili, cornbread, beans (which could later be refried for tacos), pizzas cut up into individual slices—could actually save her time in the long run. And having cut-up crunchies or low-sugar sweets like homemade oatmeal cookies within a hungry hand's reach might help wean her sugar-loving adolescents off their regular fix.

A more realistic solution, says Dr. LaChance, would be to simply supplement the family's fast foods with items to make a complete meal. "If you're eating a hamburger or a pizza, which is not such bad food, make sure you have a salad and a glass of skim milk, too, not a soda," he says.

And you can choose convenience foods with an eye toward more nourishment and less fat and salt. Look for stir-fry meat and vegetable combinations and dieter's dinners, and pick store-brand frozen vegetables without butter or sauces.

Nutritional danger zones can make an unexpected appearance in just about anyone's dietary lifestyle. But once we're aware of them, that's half the battle. And the rest, our nutritionists agree, is not that difficult.

And the Answers Are . . .

The four basic food groups are: meat and eggs, dairy products, grains and cereals, and fruits and vegetables.

Romaine has six times as much vitamin A and three times as much calcium and vitamin C as iceberg lettuce.

Brown rice has three times as much fiber and twice as much potassium and riboflavin as white rice.

Nuts, beans, whole grains and green leafy vegetables are rich in magnesium.

Bananas, oranges, potatoes and tomatoes have lots of potassium.

Meat, whole grains and nuts are good sources of zinc.

The American Health Foundation, a leading nonprofit research group, recommends you get 20 to 25 percent of your calories from fat, 15 percent from protein and 60 to 65 percent from carbohydrates.

Scientists now list between 50 and 60 known nutrients needed by the body.

CHAPTER 3

Eating for One

A popular comedienne once joked that she wanted to open a restaurant strictly for singles. Her scheme was to make them feel at home. Instead of a table, each diner would eat standing over a sink.

The image should strike a familiar chord in anyone who has ever lived alone. You know who you are. You're the ones who've made peanut-butter fudge brownies for supper, eaten cold pizza for breakfast and consumed whole meals bathed in a romantic glow of refrigerator light. The closest you've ever come to owning a pet is something in the back of the fridge with fur on it. Was that once tapioca pudding?

Needless to say, good nutrition rarely comes in single servings. If you're among the 23.2 percent of the American population living in what the census bureau calls a one-person household, it's a safe bet your diet makes World War II C rations look like health food.

"What do I usually eat?" says a 31-year-old single personnel consultant in Washington, D.C. "TV dinners, M & M's, Häagen-Dazs ice cream every Sunday night. I wouldn't eat this way if I weren't single. I wouldn't be so careless. But I want you to know I've seen the error of my ways . . . all 20 pounds of the error of my ways."

Like this reformed careless consumer, many singles atone for their dietary indiscretions only after they learn the direct relationship between their waist size and the number of aluminum single-serving pans in their trash. But the damage they do with their quickie over-the-sink meals and their fast-food feasts is far from merely cosmetic. Next to the poor, they may be the most undernourished people in America.

George Demetrakopoulos, M.D., M.P.H., is medical director of the Medical Nutrition Center of Greater Washington, D.C. Among the patients who come to him for nutritional assessments are people who should know about nutrition: employees of several of the government's top health-regulation agencies. But, he says, it doesn't seem to give them an edge if they're single. In a study of 40 single men and women between 25 and 45, he found most were deficient in zinc, folate, and B_6. The women were also deficient in calcium and were getting only 57 percent of their recommended daily allowance of iron.

"These are not typical people," says Dr. Demetrakopoulos. "These are nutrition-conscious people. They should have performed above average, but they didn't. Imagine," he says, "the ones who are not."

Though the research is meager, it seems to show that living alone is a significant nutritional risk factor even if you're nutritionally savvy. In fact, eating for one seems to be most perilous for young single women who are aware consumers and older single men who don't know their way around the kitchen without a guide.

Researchers at Auburn University took a look at the diets of 50 single professional women, most of whom usually made food lists and menu plans and avoided convenience foods. Despite those good intentions, their diets were low in calories, calcium, iron, vitamin A and thiamine. What's more, their good food habits seemed to be done in by the frequent lunches out.

In a study of 3,477 people between 65 and 74, researchers at the University of California and the University of Texas found that poor men living alone had the lowest intake of milk products, fruits, vegetables, meat, poultry and fish of any group. And they were more likely to be getting less than two-thirds of the Recommended Dietary Allowance (RDA) of protein, riboflavin, vitamins A and C, and other nutrients.

What makes singles turn to meals of tea and toast or worse? Busy schedules, dieting, lack of motivation or cooking skills, even loneliness and depression can contribute to many a meager mealtime, says the experts. And, unfortunately, there's usually no immediate retribution for bad diet that might persuade a fast-food aficionado to change his or her ways.

"Most nutritional problems don't manifest themselves right away, so it's easy to cheat," says David Ostreicher, D.D.S., professor of nutrition at Bridgeport University in Connecticut, and single himself. "If you're not getting enough vitamin A and C, you might not know until 20 years later when you develop cancer. If you're eating a diet high in saturated fats and salt—the stables of most convenience foods—you might not know until you have your first heart attack at age 50."

The problem thus stated, what do you do? "Get married," jokes Dr. Demetrakopoulos. Or, failing that, simply steal some tricks from your married friends who are following a better diet.

Cook for Four

"Never, never cook for one," says Dr. Ostreicher. "Cook for four, eat one serving and freeze the rest in individual servings. You'll be making your own convenience foods, and you'll pay less for it and will be eating better."

Make Shopping Lists

"All my married friends have lists, none of my single friends do," says Dr. Ostreicher. Why a list? First, it will make you plan your weekly meals. And it will keep you from straying into dangerous territory: the family pack of cookies that looks too good to pass up, 500-calorie-a-slice frozen pizza and the special on heavenly-hash ice cream. Needless to say, don't go shopping hungry and, advices Dr. Ostreicher, have regular shopping days so you won't be tempted to dash into the deli for a hot pastrami on the way home because there's nothing in the fridge.

Shop with a Friend

Going on the premise that everything is better with a friend, try shopping on the buddy system. Your companion will be your con-science. "If you have a companion, you can discuss what you're going to buy and make with the other person," says Dr. Demetrakopoulos. "Alone, you'll wind up buying things you'd be better off without."

Steer for the Freezer Section

Many singles have given up on fresh vegetables because they are forgotten and then grow moldy in the refrigerator before the week is up.

"Psychologically, that stops you from buying vegetables the next time," says Dr. Ostreicher.

"But right next to the frozen convenience foods you'll find plastic bags of vegetables with nothing added that are just as nutritious as fresh. You can reseal the plastic bags, so you can use what you like and freeze the rest. You don't pay more and they don't give you all that excess salt and fat."

Don't Buy Big

Those family packs and mammoth cans may be cheaper, but it's no bargain if you have to throw half of it away. If you want to buy the bigger packages, consider sharing them with a friend. And if you see a cut of meat or produce you like in a larger package, ask a store employee to repackage it.

Develop Good Eating Habits

If you have to, pretend you're eating with a friend. Would you eat a chicken leg over the sink or swig milk right out of the bottle if you had a dining companion? Then don't do it when you're alone. "Always set the table," says Dr. Ostreicher. "You decide how. With tablecloth or place mats. Candlelight might be excessive, but get into the habit of having a place setting, even if you're just grabbing a piece of fruit.

"That stops the noshing. When you live alone, you often get into the habit, when you've got nothing to do, of standing in front of the open refrigerator snacking. Always eat at the table, always with a place setting.

Make Eating for One an Experience

Lynn Shahan, author of *Living Alone and Liking It!* (Stratford Press), says her first year eating alone she became "a pretty skinny kid" because mealtime, formerly so often spent with family and friends, lost its appeal. Her solution for happier soloing at the dinner table was to buy new and interesting foods and experiment with recipes so that eating became more of an adventure.

Don't Eat Alone

Have friends or neighbors in to dinner. Start a cooking club with your fellow singles. Call your local agency on aging to find out if your neighborhood provides free or low-cost meals for older people at community centers or churches.

Or join a group like Single Gourmet, a New York-based organization that tackles the problems of eating alone by arranging for up to 100 singles to eat out together seven to ten times a month.

Co-founder Art Fischer says it will not only improve your social life and your outlook, it may also improve your digestion. "Doctors have told us that one of the problems with single people eating alone is that they not only eat all the wrong food, they eat too fast, which can cause digestive problems," says Fischer, whose group numbers 3,000 members in the New York metropolitan area. "In a group like ours, you'll spend two to three hours eating a meal that, if you ate it alone, would be gone in a matter of minutes. People tell us that they've never been able to eat garlic before without getting indigestion, but when they eat it at a Single Gourmet dinner, it doesn't bother them at all. Really, it's the single lifestyle that doesn't agree with them."

The psychological boost of having pleasant companions and good food is inestimable. "One is a very lonely number," says Effie Seaman, a writer who joined Single Gourmet after the death of her physician husband. "This gives you a reason to get dressed up and go out, wearing your finery, which is far better than sitting in front of the TV with a sandwich.

Eat Out Wisely

Ned Schnurman, executive producer of the acclaimed PBS TV series *Inside Story,* regards eating out "as a form of theater."

"Eating is one of my principal interests. I eat out 300 nights a year," says Schnurman, in his mid-50's and single. By all logic, Schnurman should be as wide as he is tall. Instead, even with his rigorous restaurant schedule, he managed to lose 25 pounds in the last few years. How? He eats out wisely. When he chooses a dinner spot to please his palate, he adjusts his other meals accordingly. A light breakfast and lunch are the perfect aperitifs to the "good saloon fare" he favors: simply grilled chicken, fresh vegetables and "a little wine . . . very little." He avoids heavy sauces and bypasses the dessert cart for fruit. "I don't think it matters where you eat." says Schnurman. "Even if you eat out as much as I do, you can make sure you're eating things of good nutritive value."

Choose Light Fast-Food Fare

"It's a real break for singles that most fast-food restaurants now have salad bars," says Dr. Ostreicher. "But if you want to have a burger, have a plain burger. Don't order the fancy burger with the special sauce. And especially don't order a cheeseburger." Almost 90 percent of the calories in cheeses and special sauces come from fat.

Consider Supplements

"People will not make drastic changes in their diets, so I recommend supplementation," says Dr. Demetrakopoulos. Most women need calcium, he says. And the majority of the patients he has tested don't get even a third of the RDA of zinc (15 milligrams). But most single people are going to have to face up to it: A bad diet can't be rescued by pills entirely. "Going to the trouble of taking supplements when your diet is grossly inadequate," he says, "is like having a nicely painted house with no windows."

CHAPTER 4

Getting Kids to Eat Right

It's not as if a parent doesn't try. It's just that it's not always so easy when Billy locks his jaw every time you try to feed him what he should eat instead of what he wants. To make matters worse, you don't even know whether (and how often!) he trades his nutritious tuna on whole wheat for a triple pack of cupcakes in the school cafeteria.

How, then, can you possibly know for sure whether he's getting the proper nutrition—at least the Recommended Dietary Allowance (RDA)?

Unfortunately, that question isn't all that easy to answer. We know, because we asked three doctors and we got three different answers—yes, no and maybe. But they were all in agreement on one thing: How well your child measures up to the RDA is totally up to you.

Understanding the RDA

Before you can best assess your child's nutritional health, you need an understanding of what the RDA is all about. The Recommended Dietary Allowance was first developed in 1943 as a guideline for establishing an adequate intake of specific nutrients for *healthy* people in particular age groups. (This means anyone with a chronic illness or metabolic disorder cannot be included in this group. They could need *more.*) Since then the RDA has undergone periodic revisions and today the Food and Nutrition Board of the National Research Council has

21

established minimum limits for 13 vitamins, three minerals, nine trace elements and three electrolytes. Does this mean your children are expected to hit 100 percent of each category every day?

"No," says Lendon Smith, M.D., an Oregon pediatrician and author of *Dr. Smith's Diet Plan for Teenagers* (McGraw-Hill) and *Feed Your Kids Right* (McGraw-Hill). "Everyone who has any kids knows that they don't eat right every day. Even though we'd like them to it's unrealistic to expect it. You should look at the overall diet. It's okay if your child doesn't get the RDA every day. But is he getting it every week?"

Another thing to remember is that getting less than 100 percent of a nutrient does not necessarily mean you will become instantly unhealthy. Scientifically, a nutrient isn't considered on the low side until your intake falls below 67 percent of the RDA and even then, a deficiency disease isn't imminent. Knowing that alone should make you feel better if a day or two doesn't measure up.

Nutrients in Short Supply

Not surprisingly, certain vitamins and minerals are more likely than others to be in short supply in a child's diet. One study conducted at the University of Washington in Seattle tested a group of healthy children from the ages of 3½ to 9 to see how they fared on the RDA for vitamins C, thiamine, riboflavin, B_6, B_{12} and folic acid—all essential nutrients in normal childhood development. While intakes were adequate for most nutrients, some of the children showed intakes below 70 percent for folic acid and B_6 (*Journal of the American Dietetic Association,* January, 1985).

Dr. Smith feels that zinc, too, a trace element that aids normal growth, is often low in the average child's diet. But it's iron, more than any other nutrient, he says, that is most commonly in short supply.

Alvin N. Eden, M.D., agrees. This practicing pediatrician in New York City and associate clinical professor of Pediatrics at the State University of New York, Downstate Medical Center in Brooklyn, says iron is a very neglected area. "I think there's a large group of children out there who are iron deficient without being anemic. For this reason I think it's important for parents to consider giving their children an iron supplement. In fact, the most important thing I tell parents is to 'think iron.' "

Of course, if children would eat liver, the biggest source of iron, there would never be a deficiency problem. Nor would a deficiency of zinc, selenium, chromium and vitamins A, riboflavin, B_{12} and folate ever occur. Unfortunately, when it comes to liver, most kids consider going to bed without *any* supper the better alternative.

Meeting the RDA

Not to worry. There are plenty of other ways to get your liver-shy kids to eat right. By including certain core foods in the diet each day, the doctors we spoke to say you'll be doing your best to help your children meet their RDA.

For breakfast, the most concentrated form of nutrition is a whole grain cereal and a fruit, either juice or whole. "Hot oatmeal with applesauce and raisins tastes great and is very nutritious," says Dr. Smith. Or, for a change of taste, try serving leftovers from last night's dinner. "There's nothing wrong with a chicken leg for breakfast," he says. "It's protein."

Our experts also suggested it's best to pack a child's school lunch rather than depend on what's being served in the cafeteria. Whole wheat bread or another whole grain should always be used on sandwiches. It provides needed B vitamins. Peanut butter is just fine but eliminate—or at least cut down—on the jelly. Instead, substitute a banana. Always include fruit in the lunch box, too. For snacks, opt for carrot sticks or trail mix (an assortment of nuts, dried fruits and raisins).

For dinner, serve a lean meat or fish, steamed vegetables and fruit for dessert. If you want to feed your kids pastry, think whole grains, and go for oatmeal cookies instead of brownies.

Allow your kids to drink only lowfat or skim milk. "Kids shouldn't drink too much milk," says Dr. Eden. "I think milk is a little overrated. Too much spoils an appetite and it's too high in fat to be good for you. Two glasses a day is plenty."

Is there anything else you can do?

Dr. Smith suggests giving a multiple vitamin "for insurance, not as a food substitute. It's good to remember that the RDA is only a minimum and an estimate at that," he says. "And keep in mind that every child is different. How each person absorbs nutrients and their degree of wellness can vary."

The ABC's of RDA's

Question: Does RDA stand for Recommended *Dietary* Allowance or Recommended *Daily* Allowance?

Answer: It stands for both. *But* it refers to two different things. We'll explain.

The Recommended Dietary Allowance refers to the official standards set by the National Research Council's Food and Nutrition Board. This RDA is based on age and sex and estimated weight. For example, the RDA of a particular nutrient for a child of 7 can differ from the RDA for a child of 14 and both can differ from the RDA for an adult. This RDA is the standard your doctor or nutritionist follows when explaining to you whether your child is or isn't eating properly.

The other RDA, the Recommended *Daily* Allowance, is actually the USRDA which was established by the Food and Drug Administration for use by food manufacturers when giving nutritional information about their products on labels. Since food labels are small, there isn't enough room to fit the Recommended Dietary Allowance for individual age and sex groups. The USRDA merely simplifies things by using just one value— usually the largest level needed by any age group or sex group (excluding pregnant and lactating women).

In short, the RDA and the USRDA both serve important purposes. One offers simplicity. The other offers a more precise estimate of your child's daily dietary needs (see table on pages 28-31).

Two Typical Menus Analyzed

There's always room for improvement, and no one knows that better than the mother of a child who prefers peanut butter and more peanut butter.

We asked pediatrician Lendon Smith, M.D., to assess a typical day's menu for two typical children—Josh Wilson, age 11, and his sister, Elizabeth, 7, who live in a suburb of Philadelphia. Menu A lists Elizabeth's intake for one day. Menu B lists Josh's. Neither meets the daily allotment for all nutrients. A computer analysis reveals that both diets are on the low side for iron and zinc. Elizabeth's diet for this particular day is also low in some of the B vitamins and Josh's falls short for vitamin A.

By making a few substitutions, adjustments and additions, Dr. Smith illustrates how easy it can be to naturally add extra nutrients to your child's diet. In fact, with Dr. Smith's revision, Elizabeth's total nutrient intake soared to over 100 percent. For Josh, his vitamin intake more than tripled. His calcium, zinc and iron levels were boosted, too. (See table on pages 26-27.)

Menu A

Menu of a Typical 7-Year-Old Girl	Dr. Lendon Smith's Improved Menu	Dr. Smith's Comments
BREAKFAST		
½ cup sugar-coated cereal with ½ cup lowfat milk ¼ cup orange juice (store brand)	½ cup Grape-Nuts with raisins and ½ cup lowfat milk 1 whole orange or ½ cup fresh orange juice	"The Grape-Nuts will provide more across-the-board nutrients (and less sugar!) and the raisins a little extra shot of this day's allotment of iron. A whole orange is more likely to have more vitamin C, bioflavenoids and fiber."
LUNCH		
1 peanut butter and jelly sandwich on a potato roll 1 package cheese and crackers 1 cup cran-raspberry juice 3 Oreo cookies 1 peanut butter cup	1 peanut butter and banana sandwich on whole grain bread Thermos of homemade soup, such as chicken noodle soup or vegetable 1 cup apple juice 3 oatmeal cookies Celery stuffed with peanut butter	"It goes without saying that a banana is a far more nutritious choice than jelly. Whole wheat bread might be a better choice to help give her more B vitamins. The thermos of nutritious soup will help fill a child up and help eliminate her desire for cookies and candy. Apple juice will help bolster this day's low iron allotment, as will the oatmeal cookies."
DINNER		
Baked ham, (about 1 ounce) Steamed broccoli, 1 bite ½ cup scalloped potatoes, made with carrots and onions ¼ cup gelatin dessert with a bit of applesauce mixed in ½ cup lowfat milk	Baked ham (2 ounces) 1 spear broccoli ½ cup scalloped potatoes, made with carrots and onions ½ cup applesauce 1 cup lowfat milk	"With the exception of the gelatin dessert, this is a decent meal, although the child may have eaten more had she not had such a large lunch or so much sugary food at breakfast and lunch."

Menu B

Menu of a Typical 11-Year-Old Boy	Dr. Lendon Smith's Improved Menu	Dr. Smith's Comments
BREAKFAST		
½ cup orange juice 2 slices 7-grain bread with peanut butter	1 whole orange 2 slices 7-grain bread with "old-fashioned" peanut butter ½ cup lowfat milk	"The fresh orange is included for vitamin C, bioflavenoids and fiber. The milk will help increase calcium. Use homemade—'old-fashioned'—spread. It doesn't contain the salt and sugar store-bought varieties contain."
LUNCH		
1 peanut butter and jelly sandwich on 7-grain bread 1 peanut butter and chocolate granola bar Raspberry fruit bar	1 peanut butter and banana sandwich on whole wheat bread Trail mix (a dried fruit, raisin and nut mixture) Carrot sticks	"As with his sister, this boy should be weaned from jelly to a more nutritious alternative—bananas. The trail mix, unlike granola, will come a long way in improving the RDA, particularly some of the B vitamins, vitamins A and E and magnesium. The carrots will help restore this day's vitamin A supply."
DINNER		
1 slice meatloaf made with lean beef 2 new potatoes made with herb butter ½ cup peas 1 potato roll 1 cup lowfat milk	1 to 2 slices meatloaf made with extra lean beef 2 new potatoes with herbs 1 stalk broccoli 1 slice whole wheat bread 1 cup lowfat milk	"A little extra meatloaf will add extra zinc and iron, which are low on this day. The butter seems an unnecessary addition of fat to this diet and adds nothing in terms of nutrition. The broccoli helps increase the calcium intake."

Recommended Dietary Allowances Translated

Nutrient	Major Functions	RDA's for Children 4-13	Comparison to Adult Dosage	Good Food Sources Children Can Love
VITAMINS				
A	Necessary for healthy skin, good vision and bone growth. Also bolsters the body's natural immune system. Believed to help guard against cancer.	Children ages 4-6, 2,500 I.U. Ages 7-10, 3,300 I.U. Boys 11-13, 5,000 I.U. Girls 11-13, 4,000 I.U.	Less Less Same as adult male Same as adult female	Cantaloupe, carrots, dried apricots, hard-boiled eggs, sweet potatoes, vegetable soup, watermelon
Thiamine (B₁)	Helps keep nervous system functioning smoothly.	Ages 4-6, 0.9 mg. Ages 7-10, 1.2 mg. Boys 11-13, 1.4 mg. Girls 11-13, 1.1 mg.	Less Less than adult male; more than adult female Less than young adult male; same as adult male Same as young adult female; more than adult female	Baked beans, oatmeal, rice, rye bread, sunflower seeds, whole wheat bread
Riboflavin (B₂)	Carries oxygen to body cells. Also helps build healthy blood.	Ages 4-6, 1.0 mg. Ages 7-10, 1.4 mg. Boys 11-13, 1.6 mg. Girls 11-13, 1.3 mg.	Less Less Less than young adult male; same as adult male Same as young adult female; more than adult female	Almonds, cheese (particularly Brie), lean beef hamburger, lowfat yogurt, milk, wild rice

	Function	RDA		Food Sources
Niacin (B₃)	Good for memory and moods. Helps lower levels of blood fats—cholesterol and triglycerides.	Ages 4-6, 11 mg. Ages 7-10, 16 mg. Boys 11-13, 18 mg. Girls 11-13, 15 mg.	Less Less Less than young adult male; same as adult male More than young adult female; more than adult female	Almonds, baked beans, dried dates, peanuts and peanut butter, sunflower seeds, tuna, white meat chicken, whole wheat bread
B₆	Helps keep immune system healthy and keeps blood clots at bay.	Ages 4-6, 1.3 mg. Ages 7-10, 1.6 mg. Ages 11-13, 1.8 mg.	Less Less Less	Bananas, filberts, sunflower seeds, tuna, white meat chicken
Folate (folic acid; folacin)	Aids in the normal functioning of the central nervous system.	Ages 4-6; 200 mcg. Ages 7-10, 300 mcg. Ages 11-13, 400 mcg.	Less Less Same	Cantaloupe, orange juice, red beets, romaine lettuce (on sandwiches)
B₁₂	Necessary for healthy blood and nerves. Safeguards against anemia.	Ages 4-6, 2.5 mcg. Ages 7-13, 3.0 mcg.	Less Same	Lamb, light meat chicken, lowfat yogurt, milk, Swiss and Cheddar cheeses, tuna
Biotin	Helps certain enzymes utilize fats, proteins and carbohydrates.	Ages 4-6, 85 mcg. Ages 7-10, 120 mcg. Ages 11-13, 100-200 mcg.	Less More Same	Black raspberries, eggs, grapefruit, milk, oranges, turkey and chicken legs, whole wheat bread

(continued)

Recommended Dietary Allowances Translated—*continued*

Nutrient	Major Functions	RDA's for Children 4-13	Comparison to Adult Dosage	Good Food Sources Children Can Love
VITAMINS				
C	Helps hold cells together. Its antiviral and antihistamine properties are believed to guard against a list of diseases, from the common cold to cancer.	Ages 4-10, 45 mg. Ages 11-13, 50 mg.	Less Less	Baked potatoes, blackberries, blueberries, cantaloupe, cherries, orange juice, strawberries, tomato juice
D	Works with calcium to build strong bones.	Ages 4-13, 400 I.U.	More	Egg yolks, milk, tuna, plenty of sunshine
E	Promotes healthy circulation by preventing formulation of clots; protects cells against oxidation; protects immune system.	Ages 4-6, 9 I.U. Ages 7-10, 10 I.U. Ages 11-13, 12 I.U.	Less Less Less	Almonds, lobster, peanuts and peanut butter, pecans, sunflower seeds
K	Essential for normal blood clotting.	Ages 4-6, 20-40 mcg. Ages 7-10, 30-60 mcg. Ages 11-13, 50-100 mcg.	Less Less Less	Broccoli, cheese, milk, watercress sandwich

MINERALS	Function	RDA	Comparison	Food Sources
Calcium	Necessary for healthy bones, teeth and muscle.	Ages 4-10, 800 mg. Ages 11-13, 1,200 mg.	Same / More	Buttermilk, cheese, ice cream, lowfat yogurt, milk, whole wheat pancakes
Iron	Essential for manufacture of red blood cells.	Ages 4-10, 10 mg. Ages 11-14, 18 mg.	Same as adult male / Same as adult female	Chicken and turkey (light and dark meat), lean beef hamburger, molasses, raisins, sweet potatoes
Zinc	Aids normal growth; sharpens sense of taste, smell and sight; aids wound healing.	Ages 4-10, 10 mg. Ages 11-13, 15 mg.	Less / Same	Chicken legs, crab, hot dogs, lean beef hamburger, oatmeal, pork chops, shredded wheat
Magnesium	Aids calcium in forming strong teeth and bones. Helps prevent kidney stones.	Ages 4-6, 200 mg. Ages 7-10, 250 mg. Boys 11-13, 350 mg. Girls 11-13, 300 mg.	Less / Less / Less than other teenage boys; same as adult men / Same as adult women	Baked potatoes, bananas, beans, molasses, nuts, oatmeal, peanut butter, whole wheat spaghetti
TRACE ELEMENTS				
Selenium	Helps keep heart and muscles sound, enhances heart health, protects immune system.	Ages 4-6, .03-.12 mg. Ages 7-13, .05-.2 mg.	Less / Same	Corn-on-the-cob, breads, seafood, shredded wheat, tuna, whole wheat pancakes
Chromium	Helps insulin control blood sugar levels.	Ages 4-6, .03-.12 mg. Ages 7-13, .05-.2 mg.	Less / Same	Brown rice, cheese, cornbread, goose, oatmeal, vegetable soup, whole wheat bread, whole wheat spaghetti

CHAPTER 5

A Nutritional Strategy to Slow Aging

The Aging Scenario. It is as familiar and predictable as the outcome of a John Wayne movie. It is human planned obsolescence. At a certain age—different for each of us—we begin to run down. Our hair drains of its color, our skin sags like melted candle wax, our hands gnarl and ache. In time, we build a battlement of medicine bottles to repel the illnesses that attack us like a ravaging horde. In the end, the invaders win.

But there are scientists who challenge the inevitabilities of aging, who believe that anywhere along the line this scenario can be rewritten, often by something as simple as diet. And they have set about to do it, beginning with one of the most critical manifestations of human aging—the decline of the immune system.

A hundred years ago, scientists discovered that as people grew older, their organ weights changed. Lungs, liver and brain weigh slightly less in an 80 year old than they do in a 20 year old. And the thymus shrinks to a mere fraction of its original size.

It was only about 20 years ago that phenomenon went from interesting to significant. That was when scientists learned the function of the thymus, a flat, pinkish-gray, two-lobed gland that nestles behind the sternum and lungs high in the chest. Put simply, the thymus distributes and nourishes (with its hormones) white blood cells, called lymphocytes, that act as the body's army against disease.

The thymus appears to be the command headquarters for an army of cells known as T lymphocytes, which, when they meet a foreign invader like a virus or cancer cell, can be stimulated to divide into larger, active cells that react with the invader and kill it. At the same time, the T cells seem to stimulate other parts of the immune system into action: the macrophages, PacMan-like scavengers that literally gobble up the enemy, known as antigens, and B cells, which the T cells encourage to produce antibodies against the antigen.

If your immune system is working at its optimum, right now the T cells in your body could be leading a battle against cancer or infection without your even knowing it.

But as we age, the thymus, at its maximum when we are teenagers, shrinks markedly, leaving us with less of the nourishing thymic hormones and fewer young T cells to replenish our aged army. The aged T cells decline in their ability to reproduce and to stimulate the B cells to produce antibodies. "As a unifying concept, what is happening is that the control of the immune system begins to decline with age," says William Adler, M.D., chief of the clinical immunology section, Gerontology Research Center, National Institute on Aging, in Baltimore.

The Role of Diet

This shrinking of the thymus and resultant decline in T-cell function is believed to be largely responsible for the increasing illness and death rates among the elderly, particularly for cancer and infection, which until now have been considered simply part of the aging process.

Fortunately, that assumption has been called into question. "There is at least a distinct possibility that some illness and abnormalities we are seeing in the immune response in the elderly may not be a part of the normal aging process, that there are environmental factors, particularly diet, that may have a causal role to play," says Ranjit Kumar Chandra, M.D., of the Health Sciences Center, Memorial University of Newfoundland.

In 1984, Dr. Chandra organized an international conference on nutrition, immunity and illness in the elderly drawing scientists from North America, Europe, Scandinavia and even Japan to St. Johns, Newfoundland, to discuss the possibilities for intervening in the process that leaves the elderly so vulnerable to disease.

One prime area of research involves the thymic hormones. Researcher William Ershler, M.D., of the University of Vermont School of Medicine, has studied the effects of the thymic hormone thymosin on human lymphocytes in the test tube. When he added a dose of thymosin to test tubes containing white blood cells who had received shots for tetanus and influenza, the elderly cells were stimulated to produce a normal amount of antibodies, something they were unable to do before. Dr. Ershler says he hopes to test thymosins outside the test tube, in elderly people inoculated against flu. But it may be some time before thymosins become the treatment of choice for the aging immune system. There may be a more immediate, self-administered treatment, says the researcher. "You may consider taking zinc," he advises, "since some researchers in immunology and aging have shown a clear benefit in the immune system, experimentally, with zinc."

The reason? The thymus is chock-full of zinc, which is essential to both protein synthesis and cell division. Since the efficient working of the immune system depends on the rapid proliferation of cells, it's not surprising that the prescription calls for zinc.

And zinc was the answer to a paradox that confronted Robert Good, M.D., Ph.D., head of the cancer research program at Oklahoma Medical Research Foundation. In his fieldwork among malnourished children, he and his colleagues noted that malnutrition was accompanied by a profound decline in immunity. Children whose calories and protein were restricted were far more susceptible to disease and infection. Yet, in well-known laboratory studies, restriction of protein and calories in animals prolonged their lives.

What Dr. Good discovered was that it was not the protein or calorie deprivation that caused the drop in immunological function, but the lack of zinc. And other researchers have found that it is possible to correct the immunological malfunction just by giving the children zinc, before correcting anything else, says Dr. Good.

Dr. Chandra, who has also done extensive field research on immunodeficiency among malnourished children, tested the immune response in a group of elderly whose diets were supplemented with zinc for six weeks. He gave them a skin test—injecting a variety of antigens largely derived from bacteria and molds into the superficial layers of their skin. In a normal healthy person, at least one of the spots should show a swollen, inflamed reaction in about two days, meaning the lymphocytes are proliferating and the immune system has swung into action. It is not unusual for many elderly people to show no reaction to the skin test, indicating their immune systems are not mobilized to fight a threatening disease. Not surprisingly, this lack of reaction is a fairly accurate predictor of death. "Those elderly individuals who are found to be anergic (non-reactive) often die in the next three to five years," says Dr. Chandra.

But zinc may be able to change those odds. In Dr. Chandra's zinc-supplemented group, at least half increased their number of responses to the skin test, indicating there was some new life in their immune systems.

The very latest research strengthens the case for zinc. A group of scientists in Italy has discovered that at least one of the thymic hormones, called FTS, is not so much affected by the shrinking of the thymus as it is by the kind of marginal zinc deficiencies so prevalent among the elderly. They noticed that children with Down's syndrome and elderly people had a similar lack of active circulating FTS and zinc. The finding intrigued them because Down's syndrome children "show at an early age normal subjective factors of aging, such as autoimmunity, an increase in leukemia, the graying of hair and cataracts," says researcher Claudio Franceschi, M.D., professor of immunology at the University of Padua, in Italy.

That led him to consider the possibility that the shrinking thymus was taking the blame for a failure of the FTS hormone. "The glands work," says the researcher, "but produce inactive molecules." Blood samples taken from the two groups turned up a substance that was capable of inhibiting the activity of FTS in the test tube. When zinc was added to the culture, it induced concentrations of FTS comparable to those of normal, healthy young people.

What Dr. Franceschi and his colleagues believe is that FTS is biologically bound to zinc, and needs it to be active and effective. Dr. Franceschi speculates that this inhibitory factor found in the blood samples was FTS hormone not bound to zinc. "When we added zinc, the hormone was able to bind itself to the zinc molecules to become active," he says.

But the clinical results speak more than the test-tube studies. When the Down's syndrome children were given relatively small amounts of zinc as a dietary supplement (1 milligram per kilogram [2.2 pounds] of body weight), the results were remarkable. "Though it's difficult to measure," says Dr. Franceschi, "the children had less infections and lost fewer days at school. We think this is directly related to the zinc."

But zinc isn't the only nutrient under current investigation. Several researchers are probing the effects of vitamin E on the aging immune system. One of them is Simin Meydani, a veterinarian with a Ph.D. in human nutrition. Dr. Meydani, a senior research associate at Brandeis University and a consultant at the USDA Human Nutrition Center at Tufts University in Boston, tested vitamin E on immune responsiveness in aged mice.

"We supplemented aged mice with vitamin E and compared the effects by measuring different parameters of immune response," she explains. The supplemented mice showed an improvement in their responses to skin tests, similar to those given by Dr. Chandra to his elderly human subjects. And in the test tube, lymphocyte proliferation was significantly improved by vitamin E supplementation.

And Dr. Meydani thinks she and her colleagues obtained those results because vitamin E inhibits substances called prostaglandins, which can significantly influence the effectiveness of the immune system. "Prostaglandins derive from polyunsaturated fatty acids and, though they're not hormones, they act like hormones. They have a lot of different functions. In the immune system, they generally have an inhibitory effect, and vitamin E appears to inhibit the synthesis of prostaglandins," she explains.

Another group of scientists in Belgium tested the effects of another potential immunity booster, vitamin C, in a group of healthy volunteers over 70. One group was treated for a month with intramuscular injections of 500 milligrams of vitamin C—many times the Recommended Daily Allowance—while the other group was treated with a placebo injection of saline solution. The group that received the vitamin C had better skin-test responses to tuberculin antigens and, in the test tube, their lymphocytes were more active when exposed to a stimulatory substance. One of the reasons for the results may be the role vitamin C plays in helping thymic hormones in their job of changing immature, inactive T lymphocytes into cells ready to battle disease, the researchers suggest (*Gerontology,* vol. 29, no. 5, 1983).

The practical implications of this exciting research are obvious. "Anywhere from 7 to 10 percent of the population of North America and Europe is above the age of 65," says Dr. Chandra. "In the year 2020 the proportion of the elderly will increase to at least 15 percent of the population. Even at present, though they constitute only about 10 percent of the population, they use up at least one-third of the health-care dollars, perhaps more. If we can make any dent in the illness of this age group, we are likely to save a considerable amount of health-care costs. My own feeling is that if we can identify those individuals who have nutritional problems that lead to immune deficiencies and can correct those nutritional problems, we can expect an improvement in immunity and also, hopefully, a reduction in illness."

CHAPTER 6

The Good Meats

Beef's been on the grill for quite a few years now. "Eat less red meat," medical researchers have said, and we've listened. Fearful of cholesterol and fat, we've switched to more chicken and fish, and heaped our salad bowls high.

And—make no mistake—you *can* eat too much meat. A diet which serves up bacon, sausage, luncheon meats, steaks, chops, hamburgers or hot dogs several times a day is a diet almost certainly too high in fat and too low in fiber to be optimally healthful.

But there's another side to the meat story. If you choose the right cuts, prepare the meat properly, and eat it in moderation, meat can be a positively health-building food.

Consider, first of all, this question. Which has more cholesterol: beef, chicken or fish? Almost everyone gets that one wrong. The answer is that they all have essentially the very same amount of cholesterol, about 75 milligrams or so to a four-ounce serving.

Second, the fat and calorie content of various cuts of beef and other meats varies from mammoth to surprisingly modest. Generalizations just don't work. Take a sirloin steak, for instance. Broil a six-ouncer as it comes out of a butcher's case and you've got 660 calories, including lots of fat. But trim away all the visible fat and you're left with a four-ounce steak that has only 350 calories. Fully 47 percent of the fat content has been eliminated.

Even more interesting, certain cuts of beef, such as round and flank steak, are quite lean to begin with. A broiled six-ounce round steak, untrimmed, has 440 calories. Cut away the ounce or so of fat on the steak and you're down to 320 calories and a very respectable fat level.

Don't make the mistake, though, of cooking meat *with* its fat, and trimming it off at the table. Some of the fat that melts during cooking will actually be absorbed into the meat. So trim before cooking, then broil on a slatted tray that permits some of the remaining fat to drip away. The result is good, lean, nutritious eating.

And, of course, if you're cooking meat that's low in fat to begin with, you're better off yet. (See table below.)

But what about *saturated* fat? Isn't beef higher in this kind of fat—believed to push cholesterol levels up—than chicken or fish? Generally, yes. But remember, generalizations can be deceiving. Choose

Rating the Beef*

Cut	Calories	Fat (gr.)	Calories from Fat (%)
Eye round	214	7	29
Chuck steak	219	8	33
Sirloin	235	9	33
Flank steak	222	8	34
Rump	236	11	40
Porterhouse†	254	12	42
T-bone‡	253	12	42
Ground beef§	248	13	47
Club steak	277	15	48
Rib eye‖	273	15	50

Sources: Agriculture Handbook Nos. 456, 8 and 8-1, U.S. Department of Agriculture.
*Figures are based on a four-ounce serving, trimmed of visible fat and cooked. Each cut provides about 35 grams of protein, about 4 milligrams of iron, as well as about 100 milligrams of cholesterol.
†Filet mignon and chateaubriand can be included in this cut.
‡Strip loin and New York strip are synonyms for this cut.
§10 percent fat by weight.
‖ Delmonico and Spencer steak are synonyms.

the really lean cuts, like round, and ounce for ounce you've got a lot *less* saturated fat than we get from such common foods as stewed chicken, peanuts, cheese, even sunflower seeds.

On the plus side, beef is an extremely good source of protein, B vitamins, iron and zinc. The latter two minerals are believed to be deficient in many diets, particularly in women who are watching their weight. And even a small amount of beef can greatly increase the amount of iron our bodies can absorb from grains, potatoes and vegetables.

However you cut it—or cook it—beef *does* have more fat than vegetables or fruits. But this is true of most protein-rich foods, including dairy products, nuts and seeds. The trick is to balance these foods with others that are extremely low in fat—fruits, vegetables, corn, rice, wheat and other grains, beans of all kinds, potatoes and pasta. Go easy on the butter and you wind up with a daily diet that includes meat but excludes excess fat.

Many health authorities recommend a diet that derives no more than 30 percent of its total calories from fat. To see how that works in practice, let's begin with a well-trimmed porterhouse steak—not an especially lean piece of meat. About 43 percent of its calories come from fat. But if you include a four-ounce baked potato, one slice of whole wheat bread, four ounces of broccoli, one pat of butter and eight ounces of skim milk with your broiled steak (a four-ounce serving), you've reduced the ratio of calories from fat to 25 percent. The total calories from this typical dinner is a quite moderate 615.

Perhaps some comparisons with meatless dishes will help you put beef's benefits in perspective:

• A macaroni-and-cheese dish, made with 1½ cups of ricotta, fontina and Cheddar cheeses, eight ounces of macaroni and one cup of milk, has about 45 percent of its calories tied up in fat. A flank steak, on the other hand, has only 34 percent of its calories in fat. In fact, most cuts of beef contain significantly less fat than comparable amounts of many cheeses (Brie, Gouda, Cheddar, ricotta, Swiss and Romano among them).

• A quiche made with two cups of Cheddar, spinach, rice, three eggs and one cup of light cream has a staggering 74 percent of its calories coming from fat. No wonder real men don't touch the stuff.

Is "Prime" Really Tops?

What can a health-conscious consumer do to negotiate the meat morass? First, familiarize yourself with the meat industry's grading system. Its top rating is "prime," which means, according to the U.S. Department of Agriculture (USDA), that the meat is "the most tender, juicy and flavorful." What makes a prime cut flavorful and juicy is fat, not only the trimable fat, but also the marbling, the flecks of fat within the lean that are impossible to eliminate. If you purchase a prime cut, it's best to cut away the trimable fat before cooking.

The meat industry's "choice" rating goes to cuts that don't quite have enough marbling to warrant the prime label. Still, these cuts are high in fat content and so should be carefully trimmed.

Ironically, as one moves down the meat industry's rating chart, one makes a healthful ascent. The "good" and "standard" ratings are given to cuts "which lack the juiciness and flavor of the higher grades," according to the USDA. The reason? There's less fat. So you have less waste, fewer calories, less cholesterol and, perhaps best of all, the healthier cuts cost less. Fortunately, the meat industry has been offering more of the leaner cuts in the market recently.

So your choices are many. Beef's gamut runs from the cuts of the loin portion, which should be consumed in moderation and in careful balance with other foods, to the cuts of the round portion of the steer, which fall within the government's 30-percent-of-calories-from-fat recommendation.

When you eat out, however, another problem arises: identifying the cuts. While most supermarkets use standard names for the cuts of beef, restaurants use many aliases, such as:

• **Chateaubriand.** This is a large tenderloin, sometimes called filet mignon. It is always at least a choice cut and it might be prime. This cut cost the restaurant more to get and it'll cost you more.

• **Surf 'n' turf.** You can ask the server wishfully if this is haddock and round steak, but typically it is a shellfish (usually lobster) and a tenderloin cut of beef that by itself would be filet mignon.

• **London broil.** This is a flank steak and a highly recommended cut at home or out. It'll cost you less in a market or a restaurant, and from a nutritional standpoint is one of the best cuts of beef.

Whether you're buying meat at the supermarket or ordering it at a restaurant, be assertive. Don't feel that you're inconveniencing the meat cutter by asking him or her to trim fat for you. And make it clear to the server that the size of the tip depends on your getting the beef exactly the way you want it. This allows you to enjoy beef, not only without reservation, but with the knowledge that you're doing something good for yourself.

CHAPTER 7

Getting the Most Out of the F Complex

Years ago nutritional scientists viewed dietary fiber the way they once viewed "vitamin B": It was supposed to be a single substance with a single function that barely got a niche in the medical mind.

But vitamin B has become B complex, and dietary fiber (the roughage of yesteryear) is now surprising a lot of people with a complexity of its own.

The American Cancer Society and the National Cancer Institute now want more fiber in our diets. The food industry embraces it. The popular press hails it. And research labs around the world add support to decade-old hypotheses that it may help prevent obesity, colon cancer, heart disease, gallstones, irritable bowel syndrome, diverticulosis and diabetic conditions.

With all this fuss it's become clear that dietary fiber is more diverse in its forms and biological effects than anyone ever imagined. And among medical people, fiber's potential for promoting health has never seemed greater. The F complex has arrived.

"Nowadays most nutritionists realize that dietary fiber is multifaceted," says Peter J. Van Soest, Ph.D., a leading fiber researcher at Cornell University. "They know that it's not just one thing, but a collection of things—a variety of elements with a variety of functions."

41

Multiple Power

This latter-day insight into fiber's true nature has already helped give the lie to some old ideas on the subject. False: "Bran" is synonymous with "fiber." False: All fiber is fibrous, or stringy. False: All fiber tastes the same.

The fallacies are more apparent as soon as you realize that dietary fiber is actually the indigestible remnants of plant cells (mostly cell walls)—remnants that come in at least six types and show up in everything from bulgur to blueberries. And the differences in physiological impact among these six classes of fiber can be as vast as that between penicillin and springwater. Here's what scientists know so far:

• **Cellulose,** the most prevalent fiber, probably comes closest to the hoary notions of what fiber ought to be. It is indeed fibrous, softens the stool and abounds in all the expected places—fruits, vegetables, bran, whole meal bread and beans.

But you'll find it in some unlikely places, too—nuts and seeds—and it does more than the old notions suggest. It increases the bulk of intestinal waste and eases it quickly through the colon. All of which means, of course, that it prevents constipation, but some investigators say that these actions may also dilute and flush cancer-causing toxins out of the intestinal tract. Research also indicates that cellulose may help level out glucose in the blood, and—because of its ability to fill you up without fattening you up—curb weight gain.

• **Hemicellulose** is a misnomer—it's not half cellulose. It has a chemical character all its own, but usually shows up wherever cellulose is and shares some of its traits. Hemicellulose, too, may help relieve constipation, water down carcinogens in the bowel and aid in weight reduction. And, like cellulose, it has no known effect on cholesterol.

• **Pectin,** though, does. In fact, it may be better at pushing down cholesterol levels than any other kind of fiber.

"For some reason, a water-holding fiber like cellulose has no influence on serum cholesterol levels," says David Kritchevsky, Ph.D., biochemist and co-editor of *Dietary Fiber in Health and Disease* (Plenum Press). "But water-soluble fibers like pectin and gums can reduce cholesterol."

But then pectin doesn't have a celluloselike influence on the stool. It can do nothing to deter constipation. Just the same, researchers have been looking into the possibility that pectin can aid the elimination of bile acids through the intestinal tract, short-circuiting the development of gallstones and colon cancer. Common sources of pectin: apples, citrus fruits, grapes, berries and—contrary to fiber lore—bran.

• **Gums and mucilages** are the sticky fibers you eat every day without even realizing it. You usually encounter them as plant-derived thickening agents in everything from ketchup to store-bought cookies.

But investigators have discovered that gums, at least, can do far more than give condiments body. They've found that locust-bean gum, karaya gum, guar gum, oat gum and others can lower cholesterol significantly. And they've shown that a few gums can even help diabetics handle blood sugar better.

"There's a lot of scientific excitement surrounding the gum fibers," one researcher says. "They seem to be more effective in the treatment of diabetics than some other fibers, and they're certainly more palatable than the water-soluble ones."

• **Lignin's** main talent is escorting bile acids and cholesterol out of the intestines. There's even some evidence that it may prevent the formation of gallstones.

You'll find high proportions of lignin in cereals, bran, whole meal flour, raspberries, strawberries, brussels sprouts, cabbage, spinach, kale, parsley and tomatoes. The more mature the vegetable, the greater the lignin content.

Going to the Source

But lignin, pectin, gum or some other type of fiber isn't exactly the kind of thing you'll find in quart jars on your grocer's shelf. Nature has already packaged them in countless foods, in combinations that can produce a startling array of physiological changes. And it's these fiber foods, not the fiber types, that researchers have scrutinized the most. Here's a rundown of fact and fable concerning some of these top fiber sources:

Bran

This flaky remnant of grains is one of the world's richest sources of dietary fiber. (Not *the* richest because the raspberry, for one, has it beat.) And it contains not one, but several types of fiber, including cellulose, hemicellulose and pectin. But the generalizations about bran can stop right there, for there are too many discrete brans, each with its own personality.

Wheat bran has a reputation for relieving constipation, and research concurs (though a recent study indicates that corn bran may be even better at solving this problem). And evidence suggests that wheat bran may help modulate glucose levels in diabetics and reduce the symp-

Finding the Fiber You Need

Fiber Type	Probable Functions	Food Sources
Cellulose	Relieves constipation, counteracts carcinogens in the intestinal tract, modulates glucose, curbs weight gain.	Apples, bran and whole grain cereals, Brazil nuts, brussels sprouts, carrots, lima beans, peanuts, pears, peas, rhubarb, whole wheat flour
Pectin	Lowers cholesterol, counters bile acids in the intestinal tract. Offers protection against colon cancer and gallstone formation.	Apples, bananas, beets, berries, bran, carrots, grapes, okra, oranges, potatoes
Gums/Mucilages	Lower cholesterol, modulate glucose levels.	Dried beans, oat bran, oatmeal
Hemicellulose	Relieves constipation, counteracts carcinogens in the intestinal tract, curbs weight gain.	Apples, bananas, beets, bran and whole grain cereals, green beans, radishes, sweet corn
Lignin	Escorts bile acids and cholesterol out of the intestines. Offers protection against colon cancer and gallstone formation.	Bran and whole grain cereals, Brazil nuts, brussels sprouts, cabbage, kale, parsley, peaches, peanuts, pears, peas, spinach, strawberries, tomatoes

toms of diverticulosis, an intestinal disorder.

A controversy is brewing, however, over whether your morning bowl of wheat bran can have a positive effect on cholesterol. Most of the evidence has said no, but the latest study on the subject begs to differ. Investigators in Sweden added concentrated wheat bran to the diets of patients with high cholesterol levels, then monitored the effects. Surprise: The patient's LDP and VLDL cholesterol (the harmful kinds) decreased slightly, and HDL cholesterol (the beneficial kind) increased dramatically.

There's no such controversy, though, surrounding the cholesterol-lowering effects of oat bran. James W. Anderson, M.D., of the University of Kentucky, in Lexington, demonstrated in several studies that adding oat bran to the diet can reduce cholesterol levels drastically. In one such experiment involving men with elevated cholesterol, the reduction averaged 13 percent.

On top of that, says Dr. Anderson, oat bran is tastier than a lot of other fiber-rich fare. "Oat bran is palatable as a hot cereal and can be incorporated into muffins, breads and other prepared foods," he says.

But it would be a mistake to expect oat bran to relieve constipation. It's rich in water-soluble fiber, which generally has no effect on bowel movements.

Corn bran, however, is more versatile, It can not only ease symptoms of constipation, but lower LDL cholesterol, reduce the blood fats known as triglycerides and perhaps improve the body's ability to handle glucose or blood sugars. This latter capability was suggested by a study indicating that a daily intake of as little as 26 grams (less than an ounce) of corn bran could improve people's scores on glucose-tolerance tests.

Legumes

Peas, soybeans, lentils, chick-peas—these and their kin have high fiber content, but few people realize just how high. They actually outdo most fruits and vegetables. Canned baked beans, for example, register over 7 grams of dietary fiber per 100 grams of bean (about 3½ ounces), while cooked broccoli weighs in at around 4, and cooked cabbage at just under 3.

Much of this fiber is water-soluble, which, as you might guess, makes legumes likely agents for lowering cholesterol. And research is slowly confirming this crucial capability. Dr. Anderson and a colleague, for example, recently discovered that they could lower serum cholesterol in men with excessive cholesterol levels by adding about four ounces of pinto and navy beans to the men's daily meals. Total cholesterol dropped a remarkable 19 percent.

"While bean-supplemented diets were as effective as oat bran-supplemented diets in lowering serum cholesterol concentrations," the investigators say, "oat bran was better tolerated [fewer problems like intestinal gas] by our patients" (*Unconventional Sources of Dietary Fiber,* American Chemical Society). But can legumes help ease the problem of constipation? Probably not. Can they help control glucose levels? Probably, especially if the legumes happen to be soybeans. Researchers have been reporting that both soy hulls and a powdered soy supplement can improve glucose tolerance.

Vegetables and Fruits

Scientists have tested very few of these for fiberlike feats of physiology, though it's obvious that these foods contain types of fiber known to do a lot of healthful deeds. Researchers instead have busied themselves with measuring the fiber constituents and total fiber content of these edibles—and overturned some misconceptions in the process.

For example, we now know that "vegetable fiber" isn't all cellulose. Often, as in the case of green beans and brussels sprouts, it's not even *mostly* cellulose. Similarly, "fruit fiber" isn't 100 percent pectin, though it usually has a high percentage of that fiber. Cellulose, lignin and other types are in the mix, too.

And, as you may already know, the total fiber content of a fruit or vegetable can surprise you. The vegetables with the biggest fiber ratings, for example, include sweet corn, parsnips, carrots, potatoes and peas. And among the highest ranking fruits are raspberries, pears, strawberries and guavas. Ounce for ounce, a peach has more fiber in it than a turnip does, cherries more than a green pepper, and carrots more than cabbage.

Calibrating Intake

So how much fiber should you be eating?

Some Africans, known for lower incidence of degenerative diseases, consume as much as 150 grams (about 5⅓ ounces) of fiber a day. Intake in Europe and North America, where such diseases are rampant, is 25 grams or less a day, with many people getting as little as 10 grams.

Experts don't suggest that Americans should match the high fiber intake of Africans, but they do agree that most people aren't getting enough fiber. Unfortunately, there's no RDA for fiber and very little data on optimum amounts. More and more researchers, though, are venturing some concrete recommendations based on the evidence that does exist. John H. Cummings, M.D., noted fiber expert in England, has advocated a fiber intake for adults of 30 grams (about 1 ounce) a day. And other investigators have echoed this suggestion.

"We really don't know what the optimum intake of dietary fiber should be," says Dr. Van Soest. It is possible to get some positive benefits from fiber at the 30- to 40-gram mark, but you have to adjust the amount of what is comfortable for your own body."

Even this amount is far more than many Americans are getting, so some authorities have been coupling their fiber recommendations with some sound advice. Increase your fiber intake slowly, they say, to give your system time to adjust, gradually incorporating a variety of fibers from a variety of naturally occurring sources.

After all, you have a vast F complex to choose from.

---

13 Tasty Ways to Fiber Up

1. Leave the peels on apples when you bake them or turn them into applesauce.
2. Roll chicken in corn bran or oat bran for oven baking.
3. Add barley to vegetable soup.
4. Make tostadas with beans instead of beef.
5. Top yogurt with bran, sunflower seeds or chopped apples.
6. Make your own breakfast granola with rolled oats, bran, raisins, slivered almonds and dried fruit.
7. Use fresh, unpeeled fruit instead of fruit juice.
8. Substitute beans for some or all of the meat in casseroles.
9. Concoct taco burgers by combining lean ground beef, kidney beans, tomato paste and spices.
10. Pop popcorn and munch away.
11. Create desserts using fresh, unpeeled fruit like peaches and pears. Try filling unpeeled peach halves with cottage cheese and slivered almonds, for example.
12. Eat potatoes with the skins on.
13. Mix cooked beans into vegetable or tuna salad and enjoy.

CHAPTER 8

Your Heart, Your Health and a Drink or Two

Arthur Klatsky, M.D., Gary D. Friedman, M.D., and their colleagues at Kaiser-Permanente Medical Center, in Oakland, California, just didn't know what to make of their findings more than a decade ago. And they still look rather puzzledly at them today.

In 1974, Dr. Klatsky, head of cardiology at the center, was asked to conduct a study to look for predictors of heart attacks. Using a computer, he would review thousands of medical exams, comparing the health histories of people who had gone on to have heart attacks with those who hadn't. Already known predictors—high cholesterol or blood pressure, diabetes, smoking, being overweight—would be controlled so they would not affect the results. Dr. Klatsky would look for new, unknown risk factors. Large-scale, open-ended statistical studies like these are called "fishing expeditions," so perhaps it's only fitting that Dr. Klatsky should open up a can of worms.

He did find a number of new predictors, but one in particular stood out. People who had reported in their medical history that they drank no alcohol went on to have about a third more heart attacks, and 20 percent more sudden, fatal heart attacks, than those who said they were light to moderate drinkers. ("Light to moderate drinkers" had two or fewer drinks a day. One drink is considered 1½ ounces of 80-proof whiskey, 5 ounces of wine, or one 12-ounce bottle of beer.)

"We were afraid of this finding, in a sense," Dr. Klatsky says. "We challenged it in every way we could think of in that first report. We really didn't know what to make of it because it had never been found before."

But since then a number of other studies have produced similar findings. In Chicago, Florida, Scotland, Yugoslavia and Israel, the conclusions are the same—moderate drinkers seem to be healthier than teetotalers. Even the well-known Framingham Study, a 24-year-long medical analysis of the residents of a Massachusetts town, was analyzed recently for links with alcohol intake and disease. A slightly lower death rate for all diseases, not just heart disease, was found in people drinking from one to nine ounces of alcohol a month. (That ranges from one 1½-ounce shot of whiskey every 15 days to a shot every other day, or from 2 to 20 bottles of beer a month.)

And that analysis found that even heavier drinkers (consuming four shots, four glasses of wine, or four cans of beer a day) died in no greater numbers than nondrinkers.

In another computer scan of Kaiser-Permanente medical records, Dr. Klatsky compared total deaths, not just deaths from heart attacks, with alcohol intake. He found that people having two or fewer drinks a day still fared best. Teetotalers and those downing three to five drinks a day had the same death rate, which was 50 percent higher than moderate drinkers. Moderate drinkers also spent less time in the hospital than either teetotalers or heavier drinkers.

An analysis of all these studies was done by Thomas Turner, M.D., former dean of the Johns Hopkins Medical School, in Baltimore, and now president of the Alcoholic Beverage Medical Research Foundation at Johns Hopkins. "In every one, the rates for cardiovascular deaths were lower for moderate drinkers than for either the low- or high-intake groups," he says.

Dr. Turner's analysis also showed a kind of "ceiling" for alcohol intake, an average amount above which deaths tended to increase. "The total death rate did not change significantly until alcohol intake reached six drinks per day," he says. "At that point, total mortality rates for all causes of death were elevated" (*Johns Hopkins Medical Journal,* February, 1981).

So does that mean a few drinks a day—possibly up to six—could actually "preserve" our health or at least not hurt us?

The numbers from these population studies would seem to indicate yes, but simply too many unanswered questions remain to say it's okay for a doctor to prescribe a few swigs or for a patient to self-administer in the hope of doing himself some good, Doctors Klatsky and Turner say. And they both recommend lower "do not exceed" levels.

"A simplistic view of alcohol as being good or bad for your heart is not appropriate," Dr. Klatsky says. "I don't think drinking should be a mainstay of heart-attack prevention. Some people simply want to find some justification to drink heavily, and there's no doubt of the serious harm that can do."

Let's take a look at the arguments pro and con for moderate drinking. First, the statistics.

Cause and Effect?

"Keep in mind that although every one of these studies shows a correlation between moderate alcohol drinking and improved health, a correlation doesn't necessarily mean cause and effect," Dr. Turner says. In other words, moderate drinkers may not necessarily be healthier because they drink. Other differences could account for the discrepancies. Could moderate drinkers be more sociable or easygoing than their nonimbibing friends, traits that would likely contribute to overall health? Or could teetotalers be physically weaker somehow? Might they avoid drinking because of health problems?

"Those are good questions," Dr. Klatsky says. "One of the basic problems remaining is whether nondrinkers are different from drinkers in ways other than that they don't drink." Most studies *do* separate former heavy drinkers from the nondrinking group. These people do have a higher death rate than lifetime abstainers.

Another problem is that these are statistical analyses, not laboratory studies, says Burton Altura, Ph.D., a physiology professor at the State University of New York's Downstate Medical Center, in Brooklyn.

"There is no scientific evidence either in controlled human studies or animal studies which shows that daily low ingestion of alcohol is beneficial to the cardiovascular system," Dr. Altura says.

True, Dr. Klatsky says. "And we may never have clinical evidence because you can't easily do those kinds of experiments over a decade with people. But the more studies that come along showing that drinkers are less likely to have heart disease, the more consistency we have. And the more likely it becomes that there really is some sort of effect."

Squeaky Clean?

One of the main causes of heart disease and heart attacks is atherosclerosis—arteries clogged by hard, fatty deposits. Some studies seem to show that the more you drink, the less atherosclerosis you have, even if you drink to excess.

In Dr. Klatsky's study of alcohol and hospitalization, nondrinkers were hospitalized more often than heavy drinkers for atherosclerosis-related symptoms like chest pain and heart attacks.

"The idea that heavier drinkers have less coronary blockage has been around since the turn of the century," Dr. Klatsky says. "Pathologists have said from way back how clean the blood vessels looked in heavy drinkers." And they're still saying that.

Researchers at Tufts-New England Medical Center, in Boston, matched postmortem cross sections of heart arteries of people who had had alcohol-related liver cirrhosis with artery sections of people of the same age and sex who did not have cirrhosis. Those with the liver disease showed much less narrowing of arteries and scar-tissue formation, even when they had other risk factors like smoking, hypertension and a family history of heart disease (*Internal Medicine News,* June 15-30, 1982).

Researchers now know that drinking alcohol raises blood levels of high-density lipoproteins (HDL's), blood fats thought to help prevent atherosclerosis and heart disease. But recently scientists have broken HDL into subgroups and found that apparently not all its forms are protective. HDL_2, the form raised by exercise, appears to be. But HDL_3, the form raised by alcohol, seems not to have a protective effect. William Haskell, Ph.D., associate professor of medicine at Stanford University, made that finding.

"You can't totally discount what appears to be a lower risk of heart disease with alcohol consumption, or that it may be due to an alteration in fat metabolism," Dr. Haskell says. "There may be other things we haven't looked at yet that may result in some kind of beneficial influence."

Research seems to indicate that alcohol can also help stop red blood cells from forming clots that can clog arteries.

Several years ago, research at the Medical College of Wisconsin in Milwaukee showed that even when they had as much artery blockage as nondrinkers, people who drank were less likely to go on to have a fatal heart attack. Since this seemed to be independent of the amount of narrowing of the arteries, and hence, of blood fats, the researchers theorized that perhaps alcohol interfered with blood clotting.

An English study supports that theory. Researchers at King's College, London, checked the rate of blood clumping in volunteers, in each case before and after they drank five five-ounce glasses of white wine, ate a meal high in saturated fats, and had the wine along with their meal. They found wine alone had no inhibiting effect on blood clumping. The fatty meal alone increased blood clumping. But when the wine was taken along with the meal, much less clumping occurred (*Thrombosis Haemostas,* vol. 51, no. 1, 1984).

Blood Pressure and Stroke

Alcohol may have another, very complex role in the cardiovascular system. It seems to affect the fluidity of cell membranes, changing the way cells absorb or release substances. One substance alcohol seems to affect is calcium, a mineral that plays an important role in blood-vessel constriction, dilation and spasm. Alcohol affects both blood pressure and the incidence of stroke, says Dr. Altura, a leading researcher in this area.

"Some very preliminary research suggests that low amounts of alcohol might have an antispasmodic, or relaxing, effect on some blood vessels, particularly peripheral vessels," Dr. Altura says. But he adds many cautions. In some studies, even low amounts of alcohol constricted heart, brain and kidney blood vessels.

Most studies show that heavy drinkers tend to have higher blood pressure than normal. In one of Dr. Klatsky's studies, men having two or fewer drinks a day had about the same blood pressure as nondrinkers. Women drinking the same amount had slightly lower blood pressure. But men and women who took three to five drinks a day had blood pressure a few points higher than nondrinkers. And those taking six or more drinks a day had up to ten points higher pressure and twice as many readings over 160/95.

One very recent finding in alcohol research, Dr. Altura says, is that binge drinking can lead to stroke. "When alcohol concentration builds up to a certain point, blood vessels in the brain can actually rupture," he says.

Links with Cancer

Evidence seems to be mixed linking alcohol with cancer.

"The major risk seems to be in abusers," says Selwyn Broitman, Ph.D., a Boston University pathology professor with a special interest in alcohol and cancer. High alcohol consumption has been linked with cancer of the esophagus and with stomach cancer.

A study of Japanese men living in Hawaii, though, showed three times the rate of rectal cancer in men drinking 500 ounces or more of beer a month. That's only 1½ bottles a day. Japanese men do seem particularly sensitive to alcohol, the researchers report (*New England Journal of Medicine,* March, 1984).

But because there seems to be no link between hard liquor or wine and rectal cancer, researchers think there must be something special in beer that is the cancer promoter. "The culprit might be nitrosamines, a by-product of hops brewing that most American beermakers now are attempting to remove from their products," Dr. Broitman says.

Perhaps the strongest link is the deadly combination of alcohol and cigarettes. Drinking on top of smoking multiplies the rate of cancers of the upper respiratory and digestive tract by as much as 2½ times compared to either alone, one study reports. This double whammy has been observed in people drinking four ounces of 80-proof liquor a day. Researchers at Fairfield University in Connecticut have discovered that the two combine to produce ethyl nitrate, a carcinogen (*Acta Chemica Scandinavica,* vol. B35, no. 7, 1981).

Shakespeare Was Right

No less an observer of human nature than William Shakespeare wrote that alcohol "provokes the desire but takes away the performance."

Alcohol, even in small amounts, can weaken inhibitions and render us more open to sexual advances, says Charles Golden, Ph.D., professor of medical psychology at the University of Nebraska, in Omaha. Dr. Golden and his colleagues found that alcohol interferes with the oxygen supply to the frontal lobe of the cerebral cortex, the thinking brain, so that it has less control over our actions.

And what about sexual performance?

Unfortunately, the only studies that have monitored sex hormone levels have been with large amounts of alcohol—at least 16 ounces of 80-proof liquor, Dr. Turner reports. "There's no doubt, though, that heavy drinking does lower testosterone levels," he says.

In women, the situation appears to be "entirely different and very interesting," reports Judy Gavaler, a Ph.D. candidate and research associate of one of the field's leading experts, David Van Thiel, M.D., of the University of Pittsburgh.

"It's very difficult to show any effect at all on female hormones," Gavaler says. In one study, where women were given alcohol throughout the day and blood samples taken every two hours, researchers actually saw an increase in the body chemicals that go into making estrogen, Gavaler says. "The only thing we know for sure is that large amounts of alcohol affect the male's ability to perform."

Other Bodily Effects

What do we know about moderate alcohol use and the brain? Not much, Dr. Golden admits. "We do know it normally takes about ten years of steady abuse for obvious brain damage." The brain actually shrinks as if in a kind of speeded-up aging process that hurts the ability to reason and react. Sometimes these effects go away when a person stops drinking. Sometimes they're permanent.

"Some people, though, whom we can't fully identify, develop damage much faster and at lower levels of alcohol than most people," Dr. Golden says. "It's not so much the amount of alcohol that matters, it's an individual's reaction to it. Brain damage could occur even with moderate drinking." People who seem to overreact to alcohol—who have extreme personality changes, blackouts or confusion with small amounts —might want to consider themselves susceptible, Dr. Golden says.

Researchers at the University of California, Los Angeles found that light social drinkers—people who said they drank an average of four times a week, typically having two or three drinks—did less well on cognitive functioning tests than nondrinkers, even when they were sober. Alcoholics usually do very poorly on these tests.

The questions now are, says Elizabeth Parker, Ph.D., one of the study's researchers, are these effects due to heavy drinking, and are they long lasting? "We want to know if these effects disappear when people stop drinking, and how long that takes."

So how much is too much?

"There's a big difference between dealing with a patient one-on-one and making health pronouncements," says Dr. Klatsky. "An individual doctor knows his patient and uses his judgment to come up with sound advice regarding alcohol use. I say that people who are already drinking two or fewer drinks a day and know they can control their intake need not change their habits. But it's much more difficult to say that people who don't drink should. Plenty of times they have good reasons they should not drink."

"I think the overriding message that has come out of these statistics is that there is a daily intake below which risk to health is minimal," Dr. Turner says. "We've developed a very simple table—if you divide your body weight in pounds by 30, it gives you the number of ounces of 80-proof liquor you should not exceed. If you divide by three, it gives you the number of ounces of beer. And if you divide by nine, it gives you the number of ounces of wine."

For a 150-pound man, that comes to 5 ounces of 80-proof liquor (about three shots), 50 ounces of beer (four 12-ounce cans), or 16 ounces of wine (about three 5-ounce glasses).

But other doctors are quite cautious. "There are just too many factors in those studies that have not been elucidated," Dr. Altura says.

Another problem is that people vary in their sensitivity to alcohol, and some are quite sensitive, especially to early liver damage.

"The problem is we don't know who the susceptible people are before the damage is done," says Charles Lieber, M.D., of the Mt. Sinai School of Medicine, in New York. By the time the first symptoms of jaundice and abdominal swelling occur, the liver disease is well along. "It's truly a silent disease, and all too often allows a false sense of security that all is well," Dr. Lieber says. Not everyone who gets liver disease drinks heavily, but most do.

There's no obvious way to tell if you're vulnerable to liver damage from even small amounts of alcohol, Dr. Lieber says. Getting sick or flushing may be signs, but no one is sure. Dr. Lieber can detect very early liver damage by biopsy, and hopes to develop blood tests that can detect damage while it's still early enough to reverse it.

In Short . . .

• People who have two or fewer drinks a day seem to have less heart disease and illness in general than people who don't drink at all.

• *But* . . . moderate drinkers may not necessarily be healthier *because* they drink. Other still-unknown factors could account for differences between these two groups.

• Even in small amounts, alcohol can cause liver and brain damage in sensitive people. It is difficult to know if you are vulnerable before symptoms arise. And in large amounts it can lead to alcoholism, a devastating disease.

• Keep in mind than many of alcohol's reported "benefits" can probably be attained in safer ways—by not smoking, and by exercising, keeping your weight down, eating a low-fat diet and other commonsense lifestyle habits.

CHAPTER 9

The Health Scoop on Ice Cream

Americans are notoriously trendy, especially when it comes to edibles. One year crepes are in, the next year it's quiche. Now the streets are paved with pasta and kiwi dishes. But through all these years of fickle food fetishes, one thing has remained constant—our unflagging passion for ice cream.

Through thick (so to speak) and thin, feast or famine, recession, depression, rainy days and holidays, Americans have consistently taken their licks and come back for more. Even now, when it seems slightly out of character for a nation whose health consciousness has recently been raised, ice cream continues to be our major frozen asset.

According to the International Association of Ice Cream Manufacturers (IAICM) in Washington, D.C.; almost 900 *million* gallons of ice cream were sold in 1983—and that's up more than 4 percent from the year before and 15 percent from 1973, with the greatest growth in the newer high-fat, super-premium ice creams.

While ice cream's popularity has almost everything to do with taste, there persists the belief that it's somehow a step above other snack foods on the nutritional ladder. And that may indeed account for its appeal among both the health conscious and the health *un*conscious.

Whichever you are, we think it's time you were exposed to the cold facts about ice cream's nutritional status, and how it stacks up against other common snack foods.

First of all, you have to know what goes into ice cream—and we're talking about store-bought varieties, not homemade—before you can level any judgment against it. Basically, ice cream is made of cream and milk combined with sugars (table sugar, corn syrup or honey), flavorings, fruits and nuts, in various proportions. To be called ice cream, federal standards require that vanilla contain at least 10 percent butterfat, and chocolate, 8 percent. Most supermarket store brands fall into this "economy" category. The more butterfat in the mix, the fancier the name—so there are upscale, premium and super-premium (or gourmet) ice creams, with butterfat levels reaching 18 to 20 percent in certain cases.

The amount of sugar in ice cream on the other hand, doesn't vary. At a desired concentration of 15 to 16 percent, sugar is sometimes the most prominent taste. "Ice cream has to be extra sweet," says Gabe Mirkin, M.D., author of *Getting Thin* (Little, Brown), "because cold numbs the taste buds for sweetness. Just let ice cream melt and see how much sweeter it tastes than when it was frozen," he says.

On a more positive note, ice cream is, after all, a dairy product and contains many of the same good things. It can boast reasonable amounts of protein, bone-strengthening calcium (though this should never be your main dietary source) and vitamin A (from 272 I.U. for a typical half-cup serving—one large scoop—of the lower fat ice cream, to 449 I.U. for higher fat ones). And it's moderately low in cholesterol and sodium.

If you read the labels, you'll also notice that some manufacturers add stabilizers—such as guar gum, carrageenan, locust bean gum (which all come from plants), and gelatin—to protect the ice cream from the temperature fluctuations known as "heat shock." These additives help prevent large ice crystals, which tend to form when ice cream is partially melted and then refrozen. Emulsifiers (such as mono- and diglycerides) help ensure easy scooping.

According to Michael Jacobson, Ph.D., director of the Center for Science in the Public Interest in Washington, D.C., "these additives never killed anybody like eating too much fat will."

Naturally, fat is about the worst thing (calorie-wise and health-wise) going for ice cream, and wouldn't you know it's the main ingredient that separates ordinary ice cream from gourmet?

If you're going to eat ice cream, choose the one that's the lowest in fat and you'll also get the one that's lowest in calories, right? Yes, but there's a hitch, and it has to do with the amount of air that's pumped into the ice cream (called "overrun"). The lower fat (economy) ones are

Nutritional Value of Ice Cream and Other Snack Foods

Product	Serving Size	Total Calories	Calories from Fat (%)	Calcium (mg.)	Protein (% of RDA for adult male)	Sodium (mg.)
Vanilla ice cream*						
Giant's Wellesley Farms—10.2% fat	½ cup	159	47	55	4.6	NA†
Acme's Econo Buy—10.2% fat	½ cup	181	46	64	5.5	NA
Häagen-Dazs—16.6% fat	½ cup	272	59	103	8.8	NA
Frusen Gladje—17.5% fat	½ cup	275	61	82	8.2	NA
Orange‡	1 fruit	62	2	52	2.2	0
Apple‡	1 fruit	81	5	10	0.5	1
Crackers (Saltines)‡	8	96	23	4	3.6	123
Pretzels‡	1 oz. (5)	117	10	6.5	5.3	1,008
Brownies (prepared from mix)§	1 pc. (2" sq.)	130	35	less than .02	1.8	95
Tortilla chips§	1 oz. (15)	145	50	30	3.6	183
Potato chips‡	1 oz. (14)	161	63	11	2.7	as high as 284
Chocolate chip cookies (prepared from mix)§	2	150	48	less than .02	1.8	95
Milk‡	1 cup	150	49	291	14.3	120
Beer‡	1 can (12 oz.)	151	0	18	2.0	25
Cheese (processed American)‡	2 slices (¾ oz. ea.)	159	75	261	16.8	609
Strawberry yogurt§	8 oz.	260	10	280	17.9	NA
Candy bar (chocolate with almonds)‡	1 (2 oz.)	302	60	130	9.3	46
Milk shake (vanilla, fast-food)"	1 as served	352	22	329	16.6	201

*Ice creams were analyzed for *Prevention* magazine by private laboratory.
†Nutritional information not available.
‡Nutritional information from USDA.
§Nutritional information calculated directly from package.
"Nutritional information supplied by McDonald's.

usually the fluffiest, so that a half-cup serving may not be satisfying and you might be inclined to eat more.

The denser or heavier (gourmet) ice creams have very little added air, and because they are so concentrated you may be satisfied with less.

Now, is ice cream really a superior snack? That depends on what you're comparing it to. Put against apples, oranges or just about any other fruit or vegetable, no. But what about other snacks? Let's add up the calories of some common snacks and see how they compare to a dish of economy and gourmet ice creams. The table on page 58 lists typical servings of popular snack foods, but if *you're* not typical, you could be getting less or more than the amounts we've listed.

For comparison's sake, we'll use the lowest calorie ice cream (159 calories per serving) and the highest (275 calories), and assume you'll be able to hold it to the average half-cup serving.

Let's start with pretzels and beer. A typical serving of both adds up to 268 calories. By adding just one more beer you've managed to tally up 419 calories.

Cookies and milk add up to a quick 300 calories, and that's if you can stop at two cookies.

If you decide on a serving of soda and chips, that's another 305 calories. You can see that in calories alone a serving of the lower fat ice cream is a clear winner. Besides, with the exception of milk, the snack foods we've mentioned don't have the nutrients that ice cream does, while they *do* contain some baddies, such as excessive salt, fat and/or sugar.

"What about a snack of crackers and cheese?" you may be asking. That's not as bad as other snacks, is it? As usual, there are pluses and minuses. How much cheese do you eat? In our table we thought that two slices of American cheese sounded reasonable. And if you cut them into quarters, you'd lay them on top of eight crackers, right? Want to wash it down with anything? A soda, maybe? Okay, you've just eaten 399 calories. That's too much food for one snack, you say? Then, let's cut it back to one slice of cheese and four crackers plus the soda. Now the total is 272, still more than the lower fat ice cream.

However, we can't forget to mention that cheese is a good source of calcium and protein. Unfortunately it's also high in sodium and fat.

But here's the clincher. You've decided to be very responsible about snacking, so you've switched to strawberry yogurt. And you're right—mostly. Yogurt is an excellent source of protein, calcium and some vitamins. Best of all, it's *very* low in fat. But even strawberry yogurt has a major drawback—sugar. And because of that, the calories mount up to 260 for an eight-ounce serving.

But what's lowest in calories may fail the percent-of-fat test. In fact, that's ice cream's greatest downfall. Look at the fat and calorie table again. You'll see that only potato chips, candy bars and cheese rate higher in percent of calories from fat. The only positive note here is that while the fat levels are unfortunately high, the amount of cholesterol is on the low side—about 30 milligrams for the lower fat varieties and 44 milligrams for the higher fat ones. (Many doctors recommend that cholesterol be kept to a maximum of 300 milligrams per day.)

Like any snack food, ice cream has its negatives and positives, too. But there are some positives—more, in fact, than many other snacks. So we're not about to tell you to never, ever put spoon to mouth again.

Instead, take a close look at your own diet and lifestyle. Are you overweight? Do your meals consist of lots of fast-food burgers and

---

Now There's Tofutti

As the name implies, Tofutti is a nondairy "ice cream" whose base is tofu (soybean curd). The brain-child of kosher caterer David Mintz of Brooklyn, Tofutti is fast becoming the latest rage. It's sold in soft-serve form (like frozen custard) and is low in calories, has no cholesterol or lactose and, most important, tastes and feels great.

Mintz told us he spent years developing the "ice cream," testing it out on his customers along the way. The final product has been so successful that Mintz has packaged the product for supermarket consumption.

The only problem is that the newer "hard pack" Tofutti contains far more calories and fat than the original soft-serve version. It still has no cholesterol or lactose, making it the dessert of choice for the 50 million lactose-intolerant people in the United States, and for those in need of a drastic cholesterol cut. But calories in the hard-pack range from 170 to 210 for a half-cup serving (not unlike real ice cream), whereas the soft-serve version has only 128.

Check the table on page 61 for the nutritional breakdown of the soft-serve and two of the flavors found in supermarkets.

french fries? Do you routinely eat sausage, bacon and other fatty meats? Is the only exercise you get drawing your chair to the table? Then adding ice cream to your diet could well help push both your calorie and fat consumption into the danger zone.

But if fresh vegetables, fruits, whole grains, chicken and fish are your mainstays, and exercise is as routine as brushing your teeth, then go ahead and enjoy your just desserts—*once in a while*. Only consider softening the blow a little by choosing an ice cream that's lower in fat. And then put less in your dish and smother it with fresh fruit, like peaches or berries.

Nutritional Value of Tofutti*

Per Half-Cup Serving	Wildberry Supreme	Vanilla Almond Bark	Soft-Serve
Calories	170	210	128
% calories from fat	48	69	45
Protein (% RDA)	5.4	7.1	3.6
Lactose	0	0	0
Cholesterol	0	0	0
Iron (% RDA)	4	4	—

*In addition to tofu, ingredients include high-fructose corn sweeteners, corn oil, all natural flavorings, such as berries and nuts, isolated soy protein and several stabilizers like those found in ice cream.

CHAPTER 10

Coffee and You

Although in recent years some scientists have considered the rich dark brew to be simmering with potential health hazards, coffee is enjoying some revisionist thinking these days. It may not be as bad as you once thought—provided, of course, you practice moderation. In fact, you might be the best judge of how "good" coffee is for you and how much is too much.

The source of controversy over coffee is its most studied (though not necessarily largest) constituent, caffeine. Generally considered to be the most widely used drug in America and Europe, caffeine is an often powerful central nervous system stimulant that, in some people can cause modest increases in blood pressure and heart rate, arrhythmias, anxiety and sleeplessness.

For most people, caffeine taken in modest amounts is a pretty harmless and pleasurable vice. "If you're a normal person, your body can cope with 300 milligrams of caffeine a day—that's about three cups of coffee," says Manfred Kroger, Ph.D., professor of food science at Pennsylvania State University and a spokesman for the Institute of Food Technologists.

He cautions, however, that coffee, which contains literally hundreds of lesser-studied chemicals in addition to caffeine, can be ambrosia to one and hemlock to another. Response to a cup of java can be as individual as fingerprints.

"I, for instance, am not a 'normal' person," says Dr. Kroger. "If I drink three cups of coffee in the afternoon, I'll be up until midnight. If I drink one cup after six, I'll be up until three. I haven't given up coffee entirely. I've learned to work around my sensitivity."

Most people do. Coffee has a way of tipping off the body when enough is enough. "It seems that if you take too much you tend not to take any more," Peter Dews, M.D., Ph.D., professor of psychiatry and psychobiology at Harvard Medical School and editor of *Caffeine, Perspectives from Recent Research* (Springer-Verlag). "Suppose, for instance, you drink coffee during a business meeting. If you start feeling uncomfortable, you stop. That's why you see so many half-drunk cups of coffee lying around after meetings in a way you rarely see half-drunk cups of soft drinks. At a subliminal level, there's an automatic stop with coffee. You don't even have to think about it."

But a lot of people are thinking about their coffee drinking—and worrying about it, since some research studies have linked coffee drinking to heart disease, cancer, even birth defects. So, here are a few answers to the most troubling questions you may have about the last of your "vices."

Will Coffee Make Me Nervous and Irritable?

It can. The most common side effects of coffee are nervousness and insomnia, and whether you experience them depends largely on how much caffeine you're getting and your individual susceptibility. You'll have to let your past coffee experiences be your guide.

"Your body will tell you," says Dr. Kroger. "People should learn to observe their bodies the way they do their cars."

Your body, like your car, can have its knocks and pings. You may be drinking too much if you're unusually nervous, restless or battling with insomnia—that's the old coffee jitters. You could also be overdosing if you're experiencing heart palpitations, diarrhea, headache or heartburn. In some people, coffee acts as a diuretic, so you may have increased urine output.

Quantitatively, excessive consumption can be considered anything over four cups of strongly brewed coffee a day, which can lead to what doctors call caffeinism. The symptoms are identical to—and are sometimes mistaken for—anxiety neurosis. Caffeinism affects as many as 1 in 10.

How caffeine affects you personally may depend on your own metabolism or whether you drink coffee on a regular basis. One of the problems researchers face when studying the effects of caffeine on humans is that it affects habitual consumers and nonconsumers quite differently, say Peter Curatolo, M.D., and David Robertson, M.D., who reviewed the myriad caffeine studies for *Annals of Internal Medicine* (vol. 98, no. 5, 1983).

For instance, when a group of nondrinkers was given a daily dose of 250 milligrams of caffeine (equivalent to about 2½ cups of coffee), these so-called caffeine-naive people experienced small increases in blood pressure, heart rate and excretion of stress hormones from the adrenal gland. So did a group of habitual drinkers—who had abstained for three weeks before the test—when they were given 250 milligrams of caffeine three times a day for a week. The difference, however, was that the habitual drinkers developed a tolerance to the caffeine long before the week was up and no longer had any untoward reactions.

Will Coffee Keep Me Up at Night?

Your metabolism—specifically how quickly your system eliminates caffeine—may determine whether coffee keeps you up at night. In a study at Jerusalem's Hadassah University Hospital, researchers found that people who said coffee kept them up consumed less coffee—explained by their bad reaction to it—and eliminated it more slowly from their systems than people who claimed coffee didn't affect their sleep.

The researchers concluded that individual metabolism dictates whether coffee will rob you of a good night's sleep or not bother you at all.

Why Do I Drink Coffee?

It may be because of the taste or because of the nice buzz it gives you, making you feel that "God's in his heaven and all's right with the world." In a Swiss study, volunteers who drank the equivalent of one cup of coffee said they felt full of ideas and "go," with greater vigor, alertness and energy. Other researchers have found that caffeine can increase reading speed without increasing errors, improve the capacity for sustained intellectual effort and lead to less aggressive behaviors. There is even some indication that coffee increases aerobic capacity, which can give an athlete more staying power.

But be forewarned: What coffee giveth, coffee may taketh away. Some people experience a poststimulation let-down that can make them as tired and lethargic as they were alert and energetic. One problem you can face if you treat coffee as more than simply a satisfying beverage is that you'll start to reach for more than you can handle just to prolong the kick.

Coffee can be mildly addicting. Any coffee drinker who's given up the beverage cold turkey can tell you about the caffeine withdrawal headache and the bouts of weariness and lethargy, which, though quite real, aren't dangerous or permanent, says Dr. Dews. "Caffeine addiction isn't an addiction in the traditional sense. It's part of your lifestyle. You become attached to that cup in the morning and you miss it when you don't have it. People are that way about orange juice. They can't even talk without their orange juice. But coffee isn't as hard to give up as cigarettes, and you're not likely to drive 30 miles in the snow for a cup of coffee."

Are There Any Long-Term Health Effects from Drinking Coffee?

Early studies linked caffeine with heart disease and cancer, but since then most of those findings have been disputed and most medical experts believe there's no clear evidence supporting them. But moderation is the key. The most recent study on coffee's role in heart disease, done at Stanford University, found that sedentary men between 30 and 55 who drink three cups of coffee or more a day may be at higher risk of developing heart disease than those who drink less coffee.

There is some indication that heavy coffee consumption, when accompanied by other diet and lifestyle factors, may increase cholesterol levels, a finding of several previous studies done outside the United States. There was no such association found when the men limited their coffee to two cups a day or fewer (*Journal of the American Medical Association,* March 8, 1985).

Are There Any Special Health Problems Coffee May Aggravate?

Coffee probably ought to be taken off the menu of people with ulcers or who have experienced heartburn or other gastrointestinal problems, such as esophageal reflux, after drinking coffee. Coffee seems to promote gastric-acid secretion. People with hypertension or heart disease who experience an increase in blood pressure or heart arrhythmias when drinking coffee should follow their common sense and switch to decaffeinated coffee or a less stimulating beverage. Coffee can cause modest increases in blood pressure and heart rate and in large amounts—more than nine cups a day—is associated with arrhythmia.

Other people who ought to exercise caution are those with anemia (coffee inhibits the absorption of iron) and people who experience panic attacks, such as agoraphobics. Researchers at Yale University recently found that caffeine produces a more pronounced reaction in people who have panic episodes than in normal healthy people.

There are also a number of studies that indicate a link between coffee and tea drinking and fibrocystic breast disease, a condition characterized by benign breast lumps. Other findings, however, have cast doubts on the association. The jury is still out, but some doctors advise women with the condition to avoid caffeinic beverages.

How Does Coffee Affect My Nutrition?

There's some evidence that coffee can inhibit the absorption of both iron and the B vitamin thiamine. In the case of thiamine, it doesn't appear to be caffeine that's the culprit but another coffee chemical, chlorogenic acid, which isn't shed during the decaffeinating process.

How Can I Enjoy Coffee without Worrying?

Although moderation is the key to coffee comfort, for some the most logical step is to switch to decaffeinated coffee. Many people can't tell the difference between "decaf" and the real thing. But if you can, you might want to stick to either instant or percolated coffee which, depending on how strong you make it, can contain less caffeine on average than drip coffee.

Adding milk to coffee won't cut down on caffeine, although it tends to slow its absorption. But café au lait, that delicious French way of serving coffee by filling half the cup with hot milk and half with dark coffee, will reduce the caffeine by reducing the amount of coffee in your cup. Substitute skim or lowfat milk and you eliminate calories and cholesterol as well.

CHAPTER 11

Health-Rating America's Favorite New Foods

When Americans sink their teeth into a yummy new food, they don't easily let go. And while not all of those foods become as entrenched in American cuisine as the hamburger, they can stay popular for a long time. But just how healthful are our new preferred provisions? To find out, we've scientifically checked out some of the latest favorite food-stuffs, including some up-and-coming contenders, with our own lab tests and research. Here's what we found.

Bagels

These doughnut-shaped rolls have peaked in popularity over the last few years. Once available only from bagel bakeries, they're now found,

---

Rating Key

X Sinful
★ Enjoy only occasionally
★★ A decent, law-abiding food
★★★ Very good
★★★★ Excellent

---

fresh-baked, in supermarkets, and even in the frozen-food section.

Tradition dictates that bagels be spread with cream cheese and served for breakfast. So we compared that format with another breakfast standby—the buttered bran muffin.

Sorry weight watchers, the bagel donates 307 calories, the muffin 162. But in the fiber department, the bagel edges out the muffin 0.75 grams to 0.61. The bagel also provides 2.43 milligrams of iron, the muffin 1.28. And the bagel has about four times the thiamine (0.40 milligrams) and more than twice the niacin (3.09 milligrams) of the muffin. But the white-capped bagel also holds 420 milligrams of sodium, 190 milligrams *more* than the muffin.

But like many foods, it's mainly what you put on the bagel that can make it a health hero or a nutritional nightmare. Remove the cream cheese and the bagel drops to 208 calories and just 336 milligrams of sodium.

Rating: ★ with cream cheese ★★plain (serve warm, but not hot)

Croissants

These renowned, flaky, crescent-shaped rolls have long been a breakfast regular in France. They've really caught on here of late, and are now available frozen and oven-ready.

In the preparation, the dough is layered with an outrageous amount of butter—so much that one cookbook warns that the fat may run onto the floor of the oven as the croissants bake unless a pan with a lip is used. Result: 233 calories per morsel. And if you serve them with butter and jam, the usual accompaniments, the fat and calories of this gastronomical delight become astronomical—323 calories and 16 grams of fat each. For comparison's sake, two slices of whole wheat toast with the same toppings have but 212 calories and only 5.3 grams of fat.

Rating: ★

Gourmet Cookies

Chocolate-chip cookies have turned into big business these days, with five major companies vying for the distinction of producing the best cookie. These cookie magnates have positioned their products in shopping malls and department stores, where they sell millions of dollars worth of the delectable disks. One brand, called David's Cookies, set us back $6.55 for one pound—more than steak! So what's the big attraction? They're fresh-baked, and contain chunks of imported Swiss chocolate. And they're free of additives and preservatives. But then, so are mom's.

To see how they stack up against homemade, we had some of David's Chocolate Chunk cookies analyzed. Surprisingly, there wasn't much difference. They had about the same amount of fat and calories per ounce as home-baked cookies. But beware: David's Cookies are colossal—over 2½ times the size of homemade. So while one of mom's may burden you with 50 calories and 3 grams of fat, one of David's cookies packs 126 calories and almost 7 grams of fat.

Of course, chocolate-chip cookies aren't exactly the snack of choice for the health conscious anyway, but if you must indulge, at least don't get carried away. If you can't stop at one, don't start.

Rating: X

Espresso

What do you get when you take dark, Italian roast coffee and force boiling water through it at a pressure of 60 pounds per square inch?

Espresso, a rich, double-strength brew that, according to the National Coffee Association, has about double the caffeine of regular drip coffee. But since it's consumed in petite 3-ounce cups instead of the usual 5½- to 6-ounce serving, you end up with about the same amount of caffeine.

Rating: ★

Chicken Wings

Once no more than a side attraction, these tasty tidbits have now hit the big time. Fried and barbecued chicken wings are being piled high and served as full-blown entrées.

Unfortunately, when you wing it, the fat and calories are also piled high. A serving of fried chicken wings (about 3½ ounces, not counting the bones) bestows 321 calories and a humongous 22.2 grams of fat. To put those numbers in perspective, a comparable serving of roasted chicken breast contains 197 calories and just 7.8 grams of fat.

Rating: X

Kiwi Fruit

At first glance this brown fuzzy fruit from New Zealand is easy to pass by on your way to the checkout counter. But don't judge it by its cover. Inside it's a beautiful bright green dotted with tiny black seeds—so pretty that slices are commonly used for garnish. But kiwi fruits have more than good looks going for them. They're high in vitamin C—89 milligrams in one large kiwi fruit, which is more than the average orange or a big fat grapefruit. Iron weighs in at a respectable 0.37 milligrams, and there's also bountiful potassium (302 milligrams). They're first-rate in the flavor department, too, tasting like a cross between a strawberry and a watermelon, with just a touch of tartness. They're a great addition to green salads, fruit salads and fruit coolers.

　　Rating: ★★★★

Goat's Milk Cheese

Goat's milk cheese has a stronger flavor than cow's milk cheese, but there's no substantial nutritional difference between them, provided you're comparing apples to apples. A goat's milk Cheddar, for instance, is equivalent nutritionally to a Cheddar made from cow's milk. However, there's so much variation among the different producers that it's still best to read the label. We found one brand of goat's milk Cheddar that's said to contain half the cholesterol of cow's milk Cheddar.

　　In addition, we analyzed chèvre, a popular goat's milk cheese, and compared it to cow's milk Cheddar, just to have a point of reference. We found that they have about the same amount of fat—31.2 and 32.2 percent, respectively. Surprisingly though, the chèvre has 40 percent less protein—4.4 grams per one-ounce serving versus 7.1 grams for Cheddar. One ounce of the chèvre provides 233 milligrams of calcium; one ounce of Cheddar provides 212 milligrams.

　　Rating: ★

Monkfish and Shark

Fish is a wonderful, versatile, healthy food, and these two are no exceptions. Monkfish showed up in recent years as thick white fillets that cook up to a consistency very similar to lobster. Its nutrient punch, however, is similar to cod, another firm white fish. And cod is a good source of thiamine, riboflavin and niacin (0.08, 0.09 and 2.8 milligrams respectively per 4½ ounces raw), yet very low in fat (only 0.4 grams), sodium (90 milligrams) and calories (a mere 100). A great catch!

The thought of shark generally inspires fear rather than hunger, but it's turning up on more and more menus lately. Its taste is similar to that of swordfish, and our analysis of broiled mako shark describes a main dish with only 0.2 grams of fat, 138 calories and 113 milligrams of sodium per serving—nothing to be afraid of.

Rating: ★★★★ (unless you drench them with butter)

Mussels

These blue-black shellfish have long been popular in Europe, but are now appearing on more and more American menus, as well as in fish stores. They're available year-round on the east coast, but only November through April on the west coast, where the presence of poisonous plankton in the summer waters taints the mussels, making them dangerous to eat.

Otherwise, bought fresh from a reputable dealer and cooked well, mussels are a healthy, low-fat protein source. A 3½-ounce serving of mussels has 14.4 grams of protein, compared to 16.9 grams for a sirloin steak. But the mussels have only 1.4 grams of fat while the steak packs 26.7 grams! The mussels also provide generous amounts of calcium and iron—88 milligrams and 3.4 milligrams respectively; the steak has but 10 milligrams of calcium and 2.5 milligrams of iron. Mussels are a real gift from the sea, and when simmered in marinara sauce, splendid!

Rating: ★★★★

Gourmet Mustards

These condiments are prepared with so many different flavorings, including herbs, green peppers and champagne vinegar, that their lineup on the supermarket shelf defies even the decision-making ability of a top executive. They're available mild and hot, coarsely ground and finely ground, and everywhere in between.

But can they do you any good? Definitely. Used in place of the usual fatty spreads, such as mayonnaise and Russian dressing, or blended into them, these sauces are a flavorful way to moisten a sandwich. So go ahead and spread 'em around.

Rating: ★★★

Shiitake Mushrooms

Sometimes called Japanese forest mushrooms, shiitake are an essential part of Oriental cuisine. Now they're available in this country, most frequently in the dried form. But that's just fine, because their flavor and aroma actually increase with drying. In fact they're so flavorful that they should be used sparingly — a little goes a long way. They're best used in soups and stews, where they impart an interesting, meaty flavor.

Rating: ★★★

Radicchio

A variety of wild chicory, this highly prized Italian-born salad vegetable (pronounced *ra-deek'-i-o*) has been making the rounds of fine restaurant menus for some time, delighting customers with its pleasantly bitter taste. The small, delicate heads are about the size of a baseball, but what makes this crinkly leaf a real standout is its color — stunning red! Its popularity has grown so much that it's now available in some supermarkets.

In fact, radicchio has become so popular so fast that our analysis is, as far as we know, the very first that's been done. Popeye take note — a serving of radicchio has 82 percent of the iron found the same size serving of spinach — 1.4 milligrams compared to 1.7 milligrams. Vitamin C, unfortunately, is only about half that found in spinach.

Rating: ★★★

Salsa

This sauce made from tomatoes, chili peppers, onions, vinegar, fresh coriander leaves and corn oil is one of the staples of Mexican cuisine. It's used on everything from tostadas to tacos — even on plain lettuce. It's usually served at the table so each diner can add it to his or her food to taste.

Salsa is a super alternative to fatty or sugary sauces. Smother your broiled fish with it and you're adding only about 20 calories. A mere tablespoon of tartar sauce, by comparison, adds 74 calories! Salt content may run high, though.

Although it's available in supermarkets in many variations, home-made salsa is smashing and simple. It's a delicious way to pick up some potassium (135 milligrams per quarter-cup serving) and vitamin A (411 I.U.), too. Use salsa to give a Mexican flavor to any food— even eggs.

Rating: ★★★

Sushi

Most people think of raw fish when they think of this Japanese speciality, but there are many other nonfish variations that are just as tasty— and a lot safer. What makes raw fish unsafe is the possible presence of parasitic worms, which can cause nausea, abdominal cramps, diarrhea and constipation. Thorough cooking kills the worms.

One of the most popular variations of sushi is called *nori maki,* or rolled sushi. It's so attractive and tasty that it can easily become the main course instead of a side dish, appetizer or snack, as it's usually served. With vegetarian ingredients, you can be assured of safety.

To make rolled sushi, rice flavored with vinegar is spread over a sheet of *nori,* a type of seaweed. Vegetables such as dried gourd, pickled ginger or cucumbers are laid in a line across one end, and the whole sheet is rolled up. The roll is then cut into pieces and arranged on a serving plate cut-side up so the diners can see the fillings.

Sushi ingredients can be difficult to obtain if there's not an oriental grocery nearby, but you can devise your own sushi dishes with equally healthy American ingredients: Avocado, broccoli, parsley, canned salmon, crab or tuna can all be rolled into sushi. Brown rice can make your sushi even more nutritious. You can even roll the ingredients in lettuce instead of seaweed for a real "Western" version.

Rating: ★ to ★★★ depending on ingredients

Gourmet Vinegars

The recent explosion of gourmet vinegars is a real boon to healthy-food cooks. Raspberry, tarragon and champagne vinegars are only the beginning. Almost every herb, fruit, seed and spice imaginable has been used to season vinegar.

Use vinegars to flavor sauces and salads in place of salt and fat. They're a great ingredient for marinades because they impart flavor while tenderizing lean cuts of meat.

Gourmet vinegars are available in specialty food stores, but some are already available in your neighborhood grocery.

Rating: ★★★

CHAPTER 12

See If You Need More C

Ⓗow can you *not* get adequate amounts of vitamin C? Its Recommended Dietary Allowance (RDA) is a mere 60 milligrams a day, and it's found in everything from orange juice to brussels sprouts.

Yet, like a lot of people, you may have a deficit of C without even being aware of it. Your body, though, will know the score. Frequent infections, wounds that take forever to heal, bleeding gums, skin problems—these and other calamities may be your body's way of saying there isn't enough C to go around.

The scarcity occurs when your personal vitamin C economy goes into recession—when your C supply is too low or the C demand is too high. Your supply depends solely on your intake. (Your body can't cook up its own vitamin C—it has to be sent out for.) And your intake may or may not be what it should be. Nutritional surveys show that many people's C intakes don't even meet the RDA. Or, to look at the flip side of the problem, the demands (the forces that can increase your need for vitamin C) may be more numerous than you think. Smoking cigarettes, taking birth-control pills, living or working in polluted air, being allergic—such factors may tax your C supply to the limit.

So how do you know if you're sliding into biochemical recession? You take inventory of your C intake and requirements, and assess how they balance out.

And that's where this quiz comes in. First, read through the 19 quiz statements and check off the ones that apply to you. Each represents a vitamin C demand—a factor that may destroy C in your system or accelerate your body's use of C or possibly indicate a need for C to help prevent a medical condition.

Second, follow the instructions in the scoring section to assess your vitamin C intake and to discover how your selected demands compare. This part can't tell you whether you're in a state of vitamin C depletion (your doctor must determine that) or how much daily C you should be getting. But it can tell you whether you have a possible vitamin C deficit—whether your C demands should be outpacing your supply. (Food sources of C appear on page 78.)

Check the Statements That Apply to You

☐ 1. I'm under a tremendous amount of stress or feel tense or anxious much of the time. (Research shows that people's need for vitamin C greatly increases in stressful situations, and some investigators report that vitamin C has reduced tension and anxiety in several patients.)

☐ 2. I take daily doses of aspirin. (Aspirin can block vitamin C from entering the bloodstream.)

☐ 3. I don't adjust well to hot or cold environments. (Vitamin C has been used to treat people with heat stress, to help workers adapt to heat and humidity and to enable people to withstand cold weather.)

☐ 4. I'm recovering from surgery or have a burn or wound. (Researchers have found that vitamin C is crucial for normal wound repair and may dramatically accelerate healing of bedsores, burns and surgical incisions.)

☐ 5. I eat a high-fat, high-cholesterol diet or have elevated cholesterol and triglyceride levels. (Studies from around the world indicate that vitamin C may reduce cholesterol and triglycerides in humans and thus help decrease their risk of heart disease.)

☐ 6. I live or work around toxic chemicals or in polluted air. (In human and animal studies vitamin C has been shown to protect the body against environmental poisons—including the industrial toxins cadmium and benzene, the heavy metal lead and the airborne pollutant ozone.)

☐ 7. I take birth-control pills. (Oral contraceptives seem to reduce concentrations of vitamin C in the body.)

☐ 8. I have an allergy. (Vitamin C has been shown to alleviate certain allergic reactions, including those brought on by ragweed pollen.)

☐ 9. I take steroids. (Studies suggest that vitamin C may help reduce the high rate of infection among those who take these drugs.)

☐ 10. I have weak immunity and suffer from frequent respiratory infections. (Researchers have demonstrated that vitamin C can strengthen the body's resistance to bacterial and viral invaders.)

☐ 11. I smoke. (Inhaling cigarette smoke may burn up large quantities of vitamin C in the body.)

☐ 12. I have cancer or have a family history of cancer. (People with higher intakes of vitamin C seem to have lower risks of certain cancers. And with laboratory animals and in the test tube, researchers have established that C is a potent antitumor agent.)

☐ 13. I'm prone to skin problems. (Increased vitamin C intake has been associated with a lower incidence of minor skin disorders.)

☐ 14. I suffer frequent urinary infections. (Vitamin C can destroy certain bacteria, including *Escherichia coli,* the most common instigator of urinary-tract infections. Thus doctors have used C to prevent these ailments in people prone to them.)

☐ 15. I have asthma. (Vitamin C has been shown to relieve some asthmatic symptoms, including attacks.)

☐ 16. I eat a lot of processed meats, smoked fish or other foods containing nitrates. (Nitrates are often added to foods as preservatives or flavoring and coloring agents. But in the stomach they can be transformed into nitrosamines, potent cancer-causing substances. Research indicates, however, that vitamin C may be able to block this transformation or at least minimize its destructive effects.)

☐ 17. My gums aren't as healthy as they should be. (Several studies suggest that the condition of the gums can actually be improved with increased intake of C.)

☐ 18. I have glaucoma. (The common element in all types of glaucoma is greater-than-normal pressure inside the eyeball. Researchers have demonstrated that oral vitamin C can often decrease this pressure, sometimes dramatically.)

☐ 19. I'm a diabetic. (Research suggests that vitamin C may be able to improve the body's handling of blood sugar. There's even some evidence that C can inhibit or prevent damage to the walls of blood vessels caused by chronic high blood-sugar levels. Diabetics should know, however, that vitamin C may interfere with urinary blood-sugar tests.)

What's Your Score?

Now you have an idea of how many factors may be drawing on your stores of C.

To evaluate the supply side of the equation, estimate your daily C intake (including supplements) for three consecutive days and take an average. The box on page 78 will help you determine the C content of C-rich foods, and nutritional food labels can give you even more data. Just keep in mind that the cooking and storing of foods can decrease their C content below established values.

This table can tell you whether you have a possible vitamin C deficit.

If Your Daily Intake Is	And You Checked	Then You Have
Low (up to 100 mg.)	At least 1 statement	A possible need for more C
Medium (100 to 300 mg.)	1 or 2 statements	Probably no need for more C
	3 or more statements	A possible need for more C
Maximum* (300 or more mg.)	5 or fewer statements	Probably no need for more C
	6 or more statements	A possible need for more C

*Certain medical conditions may respond to even higher intakes, but such high-dose therapy should be supervised by a qualified medical professional.

The Best Food Sources of Vitamin C

Food	Portion	Vitamin C (mg.)
Orange juice, fresh-squeezed	1 cup	124
Green peppers, raw, chopped	½ cup	96
Grapefruit juice	1 cup	94
Papaya	½	94
Brussels sprouts	4	73
Broccoli, raw, chopped	½ cup	70
Orange	1	70
Cantaloupe	¼	56
Turnip greens, cooked	½ cup	50
Cauliflower, raw, chopped	½ cup	45
Strawberries	½ cup	42
Grapefruit	½	41
Tomato juice	1 cup	39
Potato, baked	1 medium	31
Tomato, raw	1 medium	28
Cabbage, raw, chopped	½ cup	21
Blackberries	½ cup	15
Spinach, raw, chopped	½ cup	14
Blueberries	½ cup	9
Cherries, sweet	½ cup	5
Mung-bean sprouts	¼ cup	5

Sources: *Nutritive Value of American Foods in Common Units,* Agriculture Handbook No. 456, and *Composition of Foods: Fruits and Fruit Juices,* Agriculture Handbook No. 8-9, U.S. Department of Agriculture.

CHAPTER 13

Give Yourself the Iron Test—and Rate Your Energy Reserves

Part I of this quick and easy quiz will let you know roughly whether your weekly menu is iron rich or iron poor. It won't tell you if you're meeting the Recommended Dietary Allowance (10 milligrams daily for men, 18 milligrams for women). It's not that precise. But it will give you some idea of what kind of iron-saver you are.

Part II of the quiz tallies the risk factors that can sap your savings of this most precious metal. Needless to say, if your Part II total equals or exceeds the total from Part I (+16, −19, for example), you may have to make some dietary or lifestyle changes to avoid the penalties of iron deficiency. If your Part I score is low yet still higher than your score for Part II (+9, −7, for example), you are probably not getting many iron-rich foods in your diet and, consequently, may not be getting enough iron despite your low risk-factor score. If the scores are close (+15, −14, for example), you may still want to make some lifestyle or dietary changes that will shrink your withdrawals and boost your deposits.

Take the following quiz, calculate *two* totals (don't add them) and compare. Then read the explanation of what it all means to your health.

Test Your Iron Level

Part I—Deposits

1. Do you eat beef liver at least once a week? +3 points _____

2. Do you eat a portion of beef, turkey, chicken, fish or shellfish at least once a day? +3 points _____

3. If you answered no to question 2, do you eat a portion of beef, turkey, chicken, fish or shellfish two to four times a week? +1 point _____

Bonus: +3 points if you eat meat for three meals a day _____

4. Does your diet include a serving of any of these at least twice a week? +2 points _____
blackstrap molasses, lima beans, sunflower seeds, prunes, dried apricots, broccoli, almonds, peas, brewer's yeast, raisins, kidney beans

Answer the next 5 questions and bonus questions only if you answered yes to any of the previous questions.

5. Does your diet include a serving of any of these at least twice a week? +2 points _____
orange juice, green peppers, grapefruit juice, papaya, brussels sprouts, oranges, turnip greens, cantaloupe, cauliflower, strawberries, tomato juice, grapefruit, potatoes, tomatoes (raw), cabbage, blackberries, blueberries, cherries

6. Does your diet include a serving of any of these at least twice a week? +2 points _____
organ meats, yogurt, almonds, wild rice, ricotta cheese, Swiss cheese, Camembert cheese, Roquefort cheese

7. Does your diet include a serving of any of these at least twice a week? +2 points _____
cashews, mushrooms, pecans, bananas, walnuts, peanuts, wheat germ, prunes, sesame seeds

Bonus: Give yourself +1 bonus point each if your diet frequently includes: _____
broccoli, dried apricots, almonds

Give yourself +½ bonus point each if your diet frequently includes: _____
brussels sprouts, cauliflower, peas, bananas, strawberries, cashews, sunflower seeds, chicken, chicken livers, brewer's yeast

8. Do you take a B complex or riboflavin supplement? (no score for multivitamins) +2 points _____

9. Do you take vitamin C supplements? (no score for multivitamins) +2 points _____
10. Do you take an iron supplement? +3 points _____
11. Does your typical meal include meat, a vegetable and a food or drink from this list? +3 points _____
orange juice, green peppers, grapefruit juice, papaya, brussels sprouts, broccoli, oranges, turnip greens, cantaloupe, cauliflower, strawberries, tomato juice, grapefruit, potatoes, tomatoes, cabbage, blackberries, blueberries, cherries
12. Do you frequently cook in iron pans? +3 points _____
Part I Total _____

Part II—Withdrawals

1. Are you a menstruating woman? −3 points _____
2. Do you have a heavy menstrual flow? −3 points _____
3. If you are a woman, do you give blood twice or more a year? −2 points _____
4. Have you recently had surgery? −3 points _____
5. Do you have a peptic ulcer, colitis or hemorrhoids? −3 points
_____
6. Do you take aspirin often? −2 points _____
7. Are you on a low-calorie diet? −3 points _____
8. Are you over 65? −3 points _____
9. Do you drink a lot of tea, especially during or after meals? −3 points _____
10. Do you eat a lot of foods containing the preservative EDTA and phosphate additives? −3 points _____
11. Do you drink a lot of coffee, especially during and after meals? −2 points _____
12. Do you eat a high-fiber diet? −½ point _____
13. Are you a vegetarian? −2 points _____
14. Do you take calcium supplements? −½ point _____
15. Do you frequently take antacids? −½ point _____
16. Do you live in an area exposed to industrial pollution, particularly cadmium and lead? −1 point _____
17. Are you involved in strenuous activity, such as long-distance running? −1 point _____
18. Do you feel you are under a great deal of stress? −2 points
_____
Part II Total _____

Explanation

Part I—Deposits

1. Beef liver is one of the best sources of dietary iron, containing 10 milligrams per four-ounce serving. That doesn't mean your body can absorb all 10 milligrams. Only about 25 percent of the iron from animal sources is bioavailable—that is, absorbed by the body. Some medical experts believe many iron-deficiency problems are the result of poor bioavailability rather than low iron intake. That's why beef liver is so important: It gets high scores not only for iron content but also for bioavailability.

In fact, you'd have to eat about 8½ pounds of broccoli to get the amount of iron absorbed from six to seven ounces of liver. And there's a bonus too. Liver also contains three other important nutrients: vitamin C, riboflavin and copper, all of which enhance the absorption of iron.

2 and 3. Again, only meat and fish have that double whammy: high iron and high bioavailability. Though red meat is highest on both counts, both poultry and fish are good substitutes. Three ounces of dark-meat turkey contains 2 milligrams of iron; a three-ounce slice of white-meat chicken provides 1 milligram, but it also contains the enhancer riboflavin, which increases iron bioavailability.

Bonus: Not only do you get a hefty dose of iron from meat, its presence in a meal helps you absorb iron from other foods you're eating. You can increase your iron intake by spreading out your meat protein—not necessarily increasing the amount you eat—over three meals instead of one or two.

4. If you don't eat meat, and even if you do, you might want to consider including as many of these foods in your diet as possible. They're all iron rich, but only about 5 percent of the iron they contain is bioavailable.

But there are ways to increase bioavailability. Take a good look at the next four food lists (questions 5, 6, 7 and the bonus question). If you can design your menu around these foods, you can sometimes double or triple iron absorption from both animal and plant sources.

5. The foods listed in this question are high in vitamin C. In one study done at the University of Göteborg, in Sweden, a glass of orange juice served with a meal of hamburger, string beans and mashed potatoes increased iron absorption from the meal by 85 percent (*Human Nutrition: Applied Nutrition,* April, 1982). The same researchers were also able to boost significantly the iron absorption from a vegetarian

meal by making sure it had a high C content (*American Journal of Clinical Nutrition,* March, 1982).

6 and 7. These are the high-riboflavin and high-copper foods, respectively. Again, they're the helper nutrients that make sure you get the most out of your iron deposits.

Bonus: Why extra points for these foods? Broccoli, dried apricots and almonds not only contain iron, they contain at least two iron enhancers. The foods in the second bonus list contain iron and at least one enhancer nutrient.

8, 9 and 10. Needless to say, taking supplements of iron and the enhancer nutrients can help if you can't eat enough to boost your iron savings.

11. You may recognize this food list. These are the vitamin C foods and this is the ideal iron-rich meal: meat, iron-rich vegetable and vitamin C.

12. Cooking in iron pans permits a considerable amount of iron to be absorbed by the food. In some cases, food cooked in iron cookware can have three to four times more iron than the same foods cooked in aluminum or glass.

Part II—Withdrawals

1-6. A government survey estimates that about 93 percent of all American women eat less than the Recommended Dietary Allowance of iron. That's the first strike against women. The second is blood loss from menstruation.

Iron is used by the body to form hemoglobin in the blood to help circulate oxygen and carbon dioxide. Because of its presence in the blood, any blood loss—from menstruation, surgery, ulcers, colitis, hemorrhoids, blood donations, even minor bleeding caused by aspirin—can leach iron from your system. Though men can certainly undergo surgery, have colitis or take aspirin, they're not as vulnerable as women. Why? Because menstruation, especially heavy menstruation (such as that caused by intrauterine devices), is a regular, monthly blood loss. It's an iron withdrawal women can, unfortunately, count on. That's why the RDA for women is almost twice that for men. And women also face a strike three: a low-calorie (and often low-meat) diet.

7. Even when women aren't dieting, they simply do not eat as many calories as men, and their intake of red meat and liver is lower. Some researchers believe they would have to eat at least as much as men to get that precious 18 milligrams of iron a day.

8. Here's another rub for women. When menopause hits, it becomes much easier for a woman to get enough iron. But menopause means you're getting older, and studies have shown the risk of iron deficiency increases with age for both men and women.

9. Drinking a cup of tea with a meal, even a meal containing a large quantity of meat and vitamin C, can reduce your iron absorption by a half to almost two-thirds, according to several studies. Why? Researchers believe it's the tannic acid in tea that binds to the iron in the meal and makes it impossible for the body to absorb it. There are a number of other iron inhibitors.

10. The common additives EDTA and phosphates, which are added to soft drinks, baked goods and other foods, can prevent iron from being absorbed.

11. Though not as potent as tea, coffee taken during or after a meal can decrease iron absorption by about 39 percent.

12. Diets high in fiber can also inhibit iron absorption, so if you're taking an iron supplement, it would be best to take it well before meals.

13. Because the most bioavailable iron is in meat, vegetarians have a harder time getting the iron they need. More careful diet management—assembling a menu rich in iron-containing vegetables and nutrient enhancers—as well as supplementation might be in order for these individuals.

14. Inorganic calcium can be a potent iron blocker. Researchers have also looked at dairy products that are high in calcium, but there's no clear evidence available to include them in the risk-factor category.

15. Why antacids? They can decrease the ability of gastric juices in the body to dissolve dietary iron.

16. Cadmium and lead, common industrial pollutants, are known iron inhibitors.

17. Strenuous exercise can rob you of iron. So-called sports anemia is relatively rare and may, in fact, be more related to diet than exercise. Unless you're a very active person eating a low-calorie, iron-poor diet, you probably don't have to worry about this risk factor.

18. Stress robs us of so many things, it should be no surprise that iron is among them.

CHAPTER 14

A Consumer's Guide to the Amazing Aminos

Only a few years ago, amino acids were a ho-hum group of 22 nutrients, with an important but unspectacular role to perform as the "building blocks" of protein. Nine of them were deemed *essential* because our bodies can't make them—we have to glean them from food.

Now those same amino acids are the hottest products on the food supplement shelf. They've been dubbed "the nutrients of the 80's" and "medical foods," and a wave of publicity about their reputed powers has sent the public thronging to buy them in unprecedented quantities.

Is such a trend justified? Perhaps. Several highly respected researchers have been revealing the benefits of amino acids for over a decade, and recent work by others shows that high doses of amino acids may have an effect on hard-to-treat diseases like Parkinson's disease and herpes. Others urge caution, saying that the public should be wary of these admittedly expensive substances until more is known about their side effects. Even those who promote amino acids say that it might still be too early to use them in large quantities without medical supervision. Here's a rundown on the most frequently discussed amino acids, and some examples of their benefits and risks:

Tryptophan

Of all the essential amino acids, tryptophan is the one that is scarcest in the American diet and, at the same time, the one most investigated by nutrition researchers. A number of scientists feel that it has promise as a safe and effective nondrug remedy for insomnia and pain.

Under experimental conditions, tryptophan in doses of one gram or more has been shown to be most effective for people who suffer from *mild* insomnia and for those who take a long time to fall asleep every night. Apparently it takes the body 45 to 60 minutes to turn tryptophan into serotonin, the brain chemical (a neurotransmitter) responsible for tryptophan's effects.

Tryptophan may also be a natural painkiller, and the dentist's chair is one place where it may prove useful. The pain of a root-canal operation is significantly reduced, according to one study, if the patient takes tryptophan supplements during the 24 hours preceding the procedure. Researchers at Temple University in Philadelphia were impressed that tryptophan worked without producing the side effects associated with other anesthesia or analgesics (*Oral Surgery and Oral Medicine,* October, 1984).

In the dose levels used in most of these trials, tryptophan appeared to be side effect-free. In the root-canal study, patients were asked to take six doses of 500 milligrams each, spaced over 24 hours. In a separate study that involved facial pain, volunteers took three grams of tryptophan a day for four weeks and experienced relief. One to three grams a day seems to be the range most commonly suggested by researchers.

If you use tryptophan, take it between meals with a low-protein food such as fruit juice or bread. Tryptophan can be thought of as the smallest child at a boardinghouse table—the other amino acids (which would be present in a high-protein meal) tend to crowd it out and prevent it from reaching the brain.

Tyrosine

If we can call tryptophan the anti-insomnia amino acid, then we can call tyrosine the antistress amino acid.

When certain laboratory mice are placed under physical or emotional stress, they stop probing their environment, poking their way through mazes or sitting up on their haunches to look around. But if those mice are supplemented with tyrosine before being exposed to stress, they don't lose their natural inquisitiveness. Their bodies apparently convert tyrosine into norepinephrine, a brain neurotransmitter that is known to be depleted by stress.

Do these findings apply to people? Yes, says Richard Wurtman,

Ph.D., of Massachusetts Institute of Technology, the experiment's author. "Supplemental tyrosine may be useful therapeutically in people exposed chronically to stress," he says. The catch, however, is that only those people who are under stress would receive a boost from tyrosine. "We did not observe behavioral effects when unstressed rats were given tyrosine," Dr. Wurtman adds (*Brain Research,* vol. 303, 1984).

Tyrosine may also help fight depression, or at least magnify the effects of antidepressant medication. One of Dr. Wurtman's depressed patients "improved markedly" after two weeks of tyrosine therapy, and her symptoms returned within a week after she stopped taking the supplements.

Although individual need may vary, Dr. Wurtman considered 100 milligrams per kilogram of body weight per day an optimal dose. That works out to be about 5,400 milligrams (5.4 grams) of tyrosine a day for someone who weighs 120 pounds. In the experiment above, the supplement was divided into three separate doses each day (*Journal of Psychiatric Research,* vol. 17, no. 2, 1982/83).

One thing to keep in mind: Don't take a supplement of valine, another essential amino acid, when you take tyrosine. Valine may block tyrosine's entry to the brain.

Parkinson's disease may also respond to tyrosine supplementation, though the evidence is weak. By a series of biochemical reactions, the body can turn tyrosine into dopamine, a vital neurotransmitter that Parkinson's patients are usually low in. The tyrosine seems to work best when the disease is still in its mild, early stages (*Neurology,* April, 1981).

Lysine

Few people had ever heard of this amino acid before it was publicized in the late 1970's as a natural remedy for cold sores, shingles and genital herpes. Because there was, and still is, no safe or effective over-the-counter treatment for herpes (though there are numerous folk remedies), lysine continues to be popular with those so afflicted— especially those people who suffer frequent attacks.

The theory behind lysine supplementation is this: Researchers discovered in the 1950's that the herpes virus can't survive without a diet of arginine. Arginine, like lysine, is an amino acid, one that is plentiful in nuts, seeds and chocolate. Researchers also discovered that lysine competes with arginine, somehow elbowing it out of the way and making it inaccessible to the herpes virus. If lysine could prevent arginine from reaching the virus, the theory went, it could prevent the viruses from multiplying and setting off an active infection.

In a study published in 1983, a group of researchers polled over 1,500 people who had purchased lysine. Among those polled (whose average daily intake of lysine was over 900 milligrams) 88 percent said that the amino acid had indeed helped them. Lysine, they said, seemed to reduce the severity of their attacks and accelerated the healing time (*Journal of Antimicrobial Chemotherapy,* vol. 12, 1983).

These results have been disputed, however, by scientists who attribute them to the placebo effect. University of Miami researchers found that when they gave sugar pills to herpes sufferers and told them it was lysine, most of the patients reported an improvement. The same researchers found that 1,200 milligrams of lysine a day failed to help those people with severe, frequent herpes episodes (*Archives of Dermatology,* January, 1984).

Glutamine

Twenty-five years ago, nutritionist Roger J. Williams, Ph.D., wrote a book called *Alcoholism: The Nutritional Approach* (University of Texas Press). The regimen that he recommended for alcoholics included supplements of glutamine, one of the nonessential amino acids. Dr. Williams claimed that glutamine reduces the usually irresistible craving for alcohol that recovering drinkers almost inevitably encounter.

Many authorities on alcoholism reject the very notion that a "sobriety nutrient" exists. But others say glutamine seems to help.

"I've been using a combination of glutamine, vitamin C and niacinamide, 500 milligrams of each, one to three times a day," says Harry K. Panjwani, M.D., a Ridgewood, New Jersey, psychiatrist and a former member of the Advisory Committee of the National Council on Alcoholism. "We don't know how it works. We can only say that somehow the craving is gone. We've used it extensively and the findings have been the same in every case."

Dr. Panjwani isn't alone. Jerzy Meduski, M.D., Ph.D., a professor at the University of Southern California and a member of the task force for nutrition and behavior in Los Angeles County, also tells us that he has had success with glutamine. "The craving for alcohol seems to be the effect of an imbalance in nutrition," he says. "There is no doubt that there is a positive response to nutritional supplementation."

Valine, Isoleucine and Leucine

Maybe not today, or even tomorrow, but at some point in the future these three amino acids may become the favorite nutrients of aspiring young Arnold Schwarzeneggers. At least one group of bodybuilders in California is experimenting with a combination of the three as an alternative to dangerous anabolic steroids for the purpose of increasing muscle mass.

"There is a theoretical basis for this, but finding the right ratio between the three has been very tricky," says Robert Erdmann, Ph.D., of San Jose, California. "Some people claim they are getting good results with it. You won't see the dramatic results that you get with steroids, but this is a potentially safer and saner approach."

Although amino acids are already being advertised in weight-lifting magazines, their safety in large amounts hasn't been established. "We don't want to mislead people," Dr. Erdmann told us. "Our research is in its infancy."

Cysteine

Much has been made of the curative powers of this amino acid, which the body synthesizes on its own. While the hype has been heavy and solid proof scarce, there is some evidence that cysteine (not to be confused with cystine) has certain therapeutic value as a nutritional supplement.

H. Ghadimi, M.D., chairman of the nutrition committee at Nassau County (New York) Medical Center, uses cysteine supplements to treat his patients who are extremely overweight. He contends that there is a link between obesity and the overproduction of insulin, and that cysteine supplements—500 milligrams taken along with vitamin C at the end of a meal—somehow neutralize some of the excess insulin, which is responsible for fat production.

Dr. Ghadimi is enthusiastic about cysteine. "Cysteine is an anticancer, antiaging amino acid," he says, "because it acts as an antioxidant." Like vitamin C, he claims, cysteine protects the body from damage by oxidants—destructive molecules also known as free radicals.

Other researchers have looked to cysteine as a natural shield against the toxic effects of tobacco and alcohol. Or, more specifically, as a shield against acetaldehyde, a dangerous metabolite of alcohol metabolism, and a toxic component of cigarette smoke. In animals cysteine has been tested for that purpose in combination with thiamine and vitamin C (*Agents and Actions,* vol. 5, no. 2, 1975).

Arginine and Ornithine

The best-seller *Life Extension,* by California health consultant Durk Pearson and Sandy Shaw (Warner Books), advised readers to fight the symptoms of advancing age by taking large supplements—several grams or more a day—of these two nonessential amino acids. But the extravagant claims made for these two nutrients are not fully substantiated.

In their book, which helped spark the new wave of interest in amino acids, Pearson and Shaw argue that arginine and ornithine can help people lose weight and put on muscle by triggering the release of growth hormones. They also claim that the two amino acids can help prevent cancer by enhancing the immune response.

But doctors don't necessarily agree with these claims. In fact, arginine and ornithine supplements may not be safe if they *do* work as advertised.

"If arginine and ornithine work—if they do raise growth hormone levels—then people shouldn't use them," says Alan Gaby, M.D., a Baltimore doctor who uses nutrition in his practice. "Elevation of growth-hormone levels can cause diabetes," Dr. Gaby says. "The bottom line is that there is no solid research on the effects of arginine and ornithine, and I would like to see more studies on their safety before I would tell anyone to take them."

Safety Is the Bottom Line

The "bottom line," as Dr. Gaby puts it, is safety. Until more is known about the safety of amino acids, they probably shouldn't be used for the self-treatment of serious illnesses. At the same time, they shouldn't be taken in large amounts for long periods.

But many of those who are researching amino acids feel that it is only a matter of time before the benefits of these nutrients are fully appreciated. They believe that amino acids may eventually replace certain drugs in the treatment of diseases such as those mentioned here and potentially many others.

"The potential for amino acids is grand," one researcher told us, and another said with confidence, "In the field of nutritional supplements, amino acids are the new frontier."